GEMMA ATKINSON

THE ULTIMATE BODY PLAN

FOR NEW MUMS

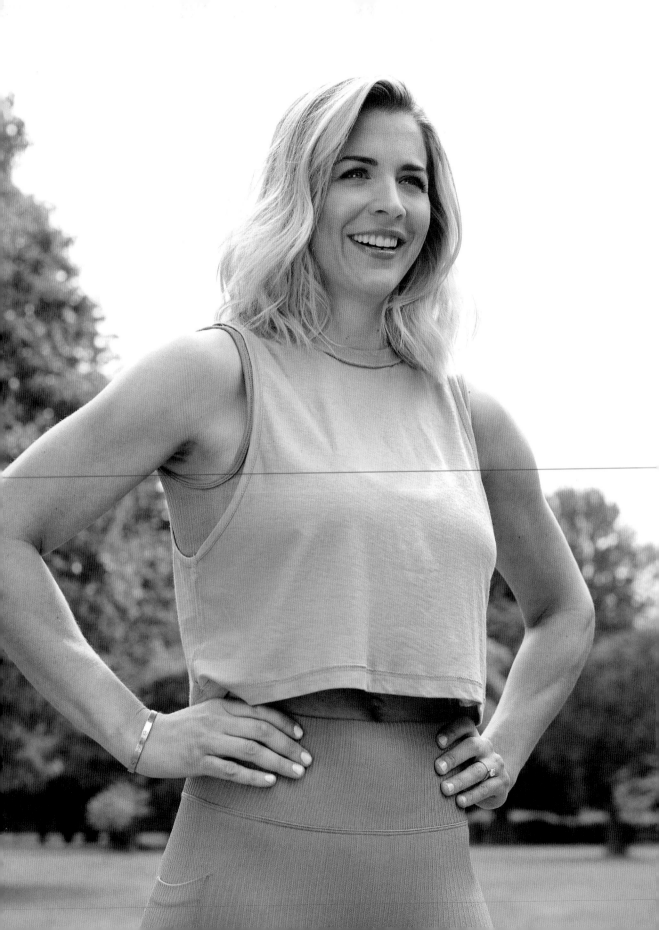

GEMMA ATKINSON

THE ULTIMATE BODY PLAN

FOR NEW MUMS

12 WEEKS to finding 'you' again

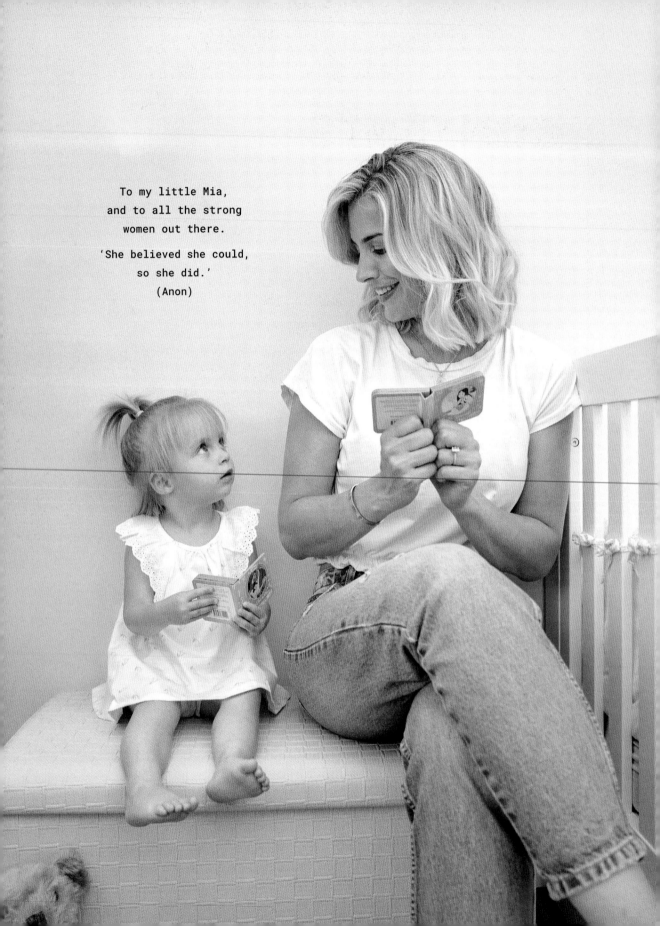

To my little Mia,
and to all the strong
women out there.

'She believed she could,
so she did.'
(Anon)

CONTENTS

DEAR READER

Thank you for picking up *The Ultimate Body Plan for New Mums*, designed to help new mums feel and look their best!

This, my second health and fitness book, contains a twelve-week postpartum fitness plan, seventy-five delicious, nutritious and speedy recipes, and also a section dedicated solely to self-care and wellbeing. *The Ultimate Body Plan for New Mums* will ensure you feel physically and mentally strong enough to handle whatever is thrown at you (probably apple purée) during this period of immense change. It's what's kept me sane ever since giving birth to my own little bundle of joy and sleep-thief, Mia, in July 2019.

At the risk of sounding like I'm at one of those cringey work away-days, I'd like to formally introduce myself: Hello, I'm Gemma. I'm thirty-seven years old, and I'm mum to Mia (as well as to Ollie and Norman, my beloved dogs) and partner to Gorka Marquez, who looks better in sequins than I do (he's a dancer, BTW, he doesn't just wear them on the reg). I love my jobs as a radio DJ, actress, presenter and model. I'm a proud Mancunian, and the strangest fact about me is that I once had a wee on the Great Wall of China next to Olivia Newton-John. Genuinely!

At fifteen years old, I was cast as grumpy schoolgirl Lisa Hunter on the Channel 4 soap *Hollyoaks*, and the rest, as they say, is history. I've worked in TV, radio broadcasting, modelling and the media for the last twenty-two years. I've travelled all over the world in different roles for different jobs, visiting everywhere from China, (see above – ahem) to the USA and Russia. But by far my biggest, most challenging and yet most rewarding job to date has been becoming a mum. Mia is the reason I decided to write this book, and I'm so happy you're reading it. Whatever encouraged you to pick it up – whether you're familiar with my work or have just had a baby and want to be able to recognise yourself in the mirror again – welcome! This plan will gently introduce, or reintroduce, fitness into your life at a pace that suits you, and it will revamp your diet for maximum energy levels.

Having a baby affects everything: your body, mind, hormones, relationships, future plans – even the state of your house, clothes and hair. I can't think of an equivalent life choice that has the same all-encompassing impact, so it's natural to feel overwhelmed and find yourself wondering, 'Wait, who am I meant to be today again?' To be clear: this is absolutely NOT a 'get your body back' plan. I assure you that the phrase 'snapping back' does not appear within these pages in anything other than an angry way. This is a 'feel stronger, healthier and more confident' plan. By dedicating just twelve weeks to training sensibly, eating well and being kind to yourself, I promise you will not only feel like *you* again, but also be more able to handle your shit (and your baby's shit – literally. TMI?).

I couldn't be more proud or excited to take you on this journey. Good luck!

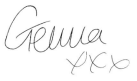

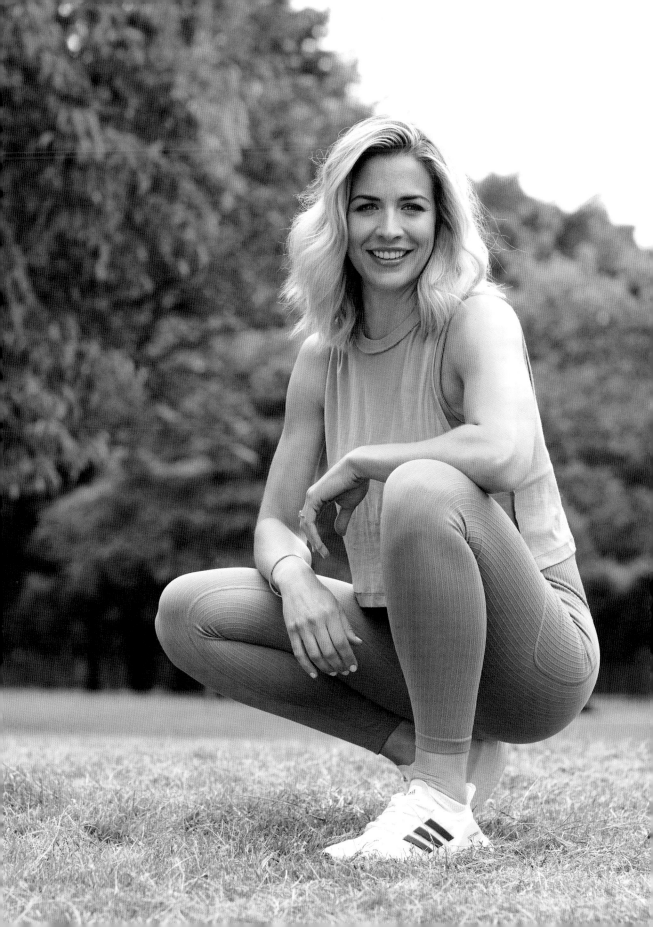

GLOW?
WHAT GLOW?

'Come on then, where the hell is this famous "pregnancy glow" everyone's always talking about?'

I was standing in front of my big bathroom mirror wearing just a sports bra and knickers, with a pile of discarded clothes on the floor next to me. It was late May 2019, I was seven months pregnant during one of the hottest Mays since records began (true – feel free to google it), and I couldn't recall ever feeling more uncomfortable or hotter (not in a sexy way) in my life. I wiped my sticky forehead and peered at my reflection more closely – or as close as I could get with my huge bump and boobs in the way.

I was looking for '*the Glow*'. You know the one I'm talking about: where your skin looks all dewy and flushed with health (not fever) and people stop you in the street to gasp, 'Wow! Doesn't pregnancy suit you!' and you laugh off the compliment modestly, knowing that, yes, in fact, you've never looked more radiant. The Glow is believed to be a result of hormonal changes: an increase in oestrogen and progesterone that gives skin a 'rosy' appearance. Increased cell turnover means knackered old cells are replaced faster, and skin looks super fresh and smooth. Not all women experience the Glow, it turns out. In fact, the hormonal changes can also cause pregnancy acne and other less-than-joyful issues, which, on top of the nausea and tiredness often associated with pregnancy, might well mean that 'glowing' is the last thing you feel like you're doing!

But I'd been really looking forward to it. Yet... nothing. Not for seven whole months. I'd had seven months of my body changing in ways I'd never dreamed of. Seven months of cramps and sweats and cravings, and not even being able to shave myself. The least I deserved, I thought, was a sodding glow. Oh, don't get me wrong, I had a glow all right – of pure sweat. My head was sweating (I don't mean just my face but my entire head), my back was sweating and, if I'm completely honest, my tits were sweating.

'The joys of having a baby,' I muttered to myself. 'You don't see this on Instagram or magazine covers.'

The least I deserved was a sodding glow.

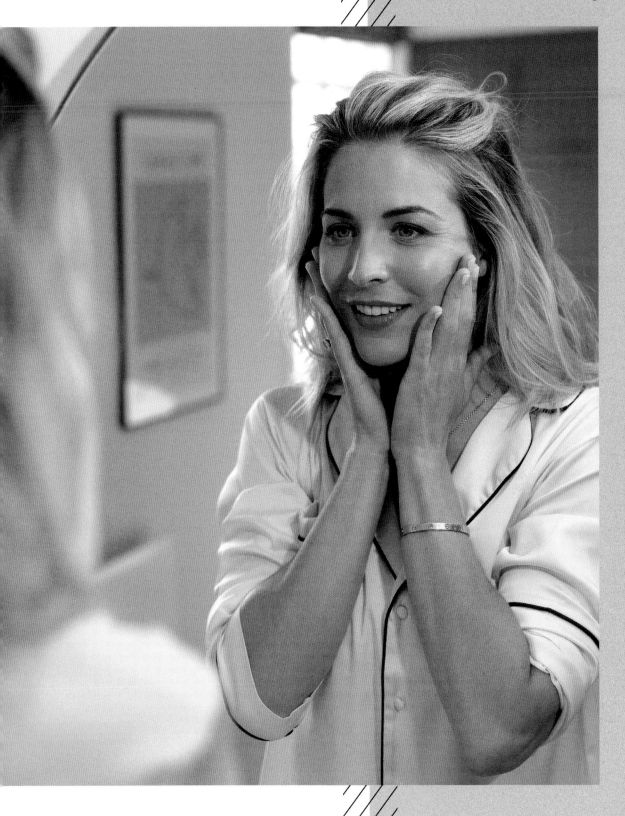

The Ultimate Body Plan for New Mums

WHY I'M WRITING THIS BOOK

Looking after yourself is always important, but never more so than when you're expecting a baby or have recently given birth. You'll discover amazing – and awful – things about your body, about your expectations of your body and about your self-esteem.

When you become a parent, everything suddenly seems beautiful and terrifying in equal measure. And, on top of the mental and physical self-reflection, you've only gone and thrown a live grenade into your home. A screaming, crying and incredibly demanding (but cute) grenade. Goodbye sleep! Goodbye showers! Goodbye sexy knickers!

Some days, you'll feel like you don't even have time to breathe. Other days, you'll feel like a fraud. And occasionally (very rarely), you'll wonder what other mums are moaning about. But, throughout it all, you'll feel better able to handle the madness if you're healthy, both physically and mentally – and the two go hand-in-hand. Looking after your body will have a direct, knock-on positive effect on your mind, and vice versa.

A lot of parenting books seem to say everything is going to be either wonderful – all flowers and unicorns – or total crap. However, my experience has been that motherhood slides up and down a constantly moving scale. Being a new mum means massive highs and big lows, and days of not much at all. I want to give women realistic guidance and advice on how to negotiate that from what I know has helped me: exercising, eating well and being kind to myself. It's like putting on your own life jacket first before helping anyone else with theirs. You'll be a better parent if you're feeling strong AF.

As I said in the welcome note, this is NOT JUST A WEIGHT-LOSS BOOK. The last thing new mums need is to be told they should lose 10lb in a month, or anything like that. This book is about how to feel strong for you and your baby, inside and out, so you can best care for your new family. It's about learning to stop comparing yourself to others and accepting that it's not about looking a certain way: it's about building self-esteem, prioritising yourself and feeling like Xena Warrior Princess (millennials may need to google that reference, but it'll be worth it).

I train and eat well because it makes me feel amazing, NOT because it makes me look a certain way. I care more about what my body can do than what it looks like – and what your body can do once you start treating it right is extraordinary.

I have spent over twenty years in the public eye and, while I am incredibly proud of and grateful for my career, being a woman working in the entertainment industry means having your appearance scrutinised every single goddamn day. I'll be honest, that's not always been easy (understatement of the decade). So, a few years ago, I decided to take control over how I felt about my body. I can't control how the newspapers, magazines or social-media trolls feel about it, but I absolutely can control how *I* feel about it.

I took up training and eating healthily and it changed my life. A real 'Eureka!' moment came in 2014 (readers of my first book will remember this story) when my personal trainer and friend, Olly Foster, asked me who in the world I most wanted to look like. I immediately replied 'Kylie Minogue!' But, instead of promising to make me look like my idol, Olly actually snorted. 'You're NEVER going to look like Kylie Minogue!' he said. 'She's five foot, and you're five-nine. You probably looked like her when you were twelve years old. Let's be realistic.' I was mortally offended. Even more so when he then flagged up how we could utilise my strong thighs (or 'thunder thighs' as they'd been called at school) and add more weights to my leg workouts. Nowwaitjustaminute...

For the first time in my life, I was being told to celebrate all the bits of my body that I'd spent years trying to hide and minimise. The things I was insecure about – my legs, broad shoulders and height – were things he was telling me to embrace and to use. It was like one of those scenes in a movie where a spotlight from the heavens illuminates the narrator, who is in the midst of a life-changing revelation.

Olly was right: I could never look like Kylie Minogue, but I could damn well look like the best version of me. I had been actively working against my body, punishing it for not being something it could never actually be. I'd been trying to make myself less, when the whole time I should have been building on and embracing what I already had – making myself more.

Since then, I've never looked back. I started training in ways that would maximise my strengths and, in doing so, I learned to appreciate my body. I felt healthier, happier and more energetic. My skin became clearer, my eyes brighter, my nails and hair stronger and I slept like a baby (a ridiculous phrase, bearing in mind what I now know). Above all, though, my confidence levels rocketed. I started not giving a f*** about what strangers thought of me, instead prioritising myself and the people I love. I was able to recognise toxic situations and acknowledge that I deserved better.

I train and eat well because it makes me feel amazing, NOT because it makes me look a certain way.

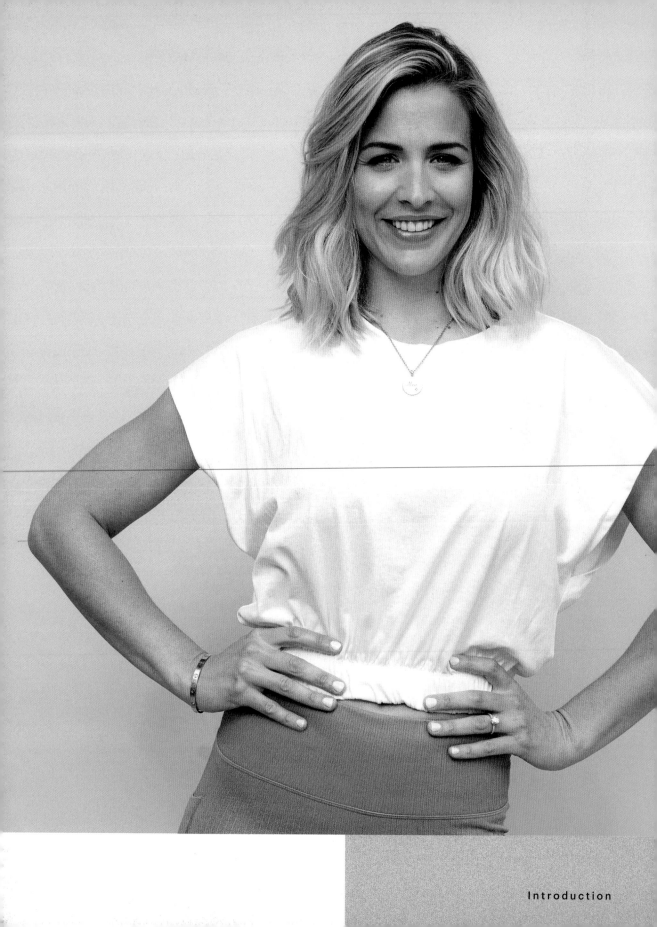

Accepting yourself and appreciating your body is more important than ever when you've had a baby. Your body has done something extraordinary, yet instead of constantly high-fiving ourselves for having BIRTHED AN ACTUAL HUMAN, we're made to feel ashamed of our pooches, stretch marks and cellulite. We're bombarded with congratulatory images of new mums who have 'snapped back' after giving birth. 'Sharon's got her pre-baby body back,' the headlines scream. Back from where? Her body didn't go anywhere! It's like carrying a handbag around filled with loads of paperwork, then, when you take the paperwork out, saying, 'Great, I've got my handbag back!' Wait, what? Your bag was still there – it was just doing a job. And it did it fantastically, thanks very much.

So, that's why I'm writing this book. To prove that training and eating right will make you appreciate your body so much more. It's about showing it some love and treating it right, in a safe and compassionate way. It took me six months to be able to get back to my pre-pregnancy training regime safely and I'm a fitness fanatic – my body was primed to get back into the gym. So imagine how long it'll take someone who doesn't train regularly and isn't familiar with nutrition to feel and look their best. Comparing yourself and feeling a failure for not looking the same as someone else is madness. It's so important to me that you're committing to this plan to feel and look better on your own terms, not because you feel you should or because someone else is putting you under pressure. The only way to stay motivated is to choose to do this for you and your new baby.

Accepting yourself and appreciating your body is more important than ever when you've had a baby.

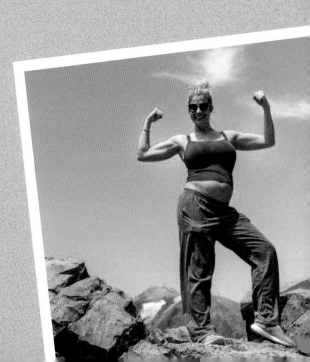

A personal challenge

I'm hoping you'll embrace this plan as a new challenge, like I did. I'd never been as big, unfit or knackered as I was after giving birth, but I'd also never had access to so much information on how to feel better. In late August 2019, a month or so after having Mia, I was asked if I'd film the *Strictly Come Dancing* Christmas special that November, dancing a jive with Gorka. A jive, of all things! What's wrong with a slow, romantic waltz, FFS? I was so tempted to say no. That would only be four months after my caesarean, and I knew I wouldn't be in the kind of shape I was used to. But then I thought about how wonderful it would be for Mia to see her mum and dad dancing together on the TV, and what an ace challenge it would be for me – both physically and mentally. I do love a transformation story; this time it would be my own! So I did it. And yes, when the time came, I was a bit heavier and definitely more tired than I would have liked, but I look back now and wonder what on earth I was worried about. I looked fantastic and was so proud of myself. I'd gone from sitting on my arse for sixteen hours a day to jiving on TV!

It's commonly known that there is a direct correlation between exercising and better mental health – and that's always been true for me. It's not only from the endorphins and serotonin released, but the fact you're giving yourself some 'me time' – something that's no doubt in incredibly short supply when you have a new baby. That's why choosing to dedicate time to this plan is a really big deal. You're telling yourself you deserve to feel better. You're investing in your own self-worth – and that's something to be proud of.

Whatever stage you're at right now, we'll have you up and doing a jive soon enough. (And, with your newly strengthened pelvic floor, courtesy of the exercise plan, you won't piss yourself during it, either!) While this is designed as a twelve-week plan, it can take as long as you like. There's no time pressure. This is a lifestyle change, not a quick fix. I want you to enjoy it! It's exciting seeing what your body can do, as long as you're doing it for the right reasons (for yourself) and in the right way.

Everyone is welcome! (Not just new mums.)

While tailored to new mums, this training programme will actually help anyone, whatever age or gender, to feel their best. Because it's been designed for people who are taking training slowly and gently, it will be particularly useful for those who are either introducing fitness into their lives properly for the first time, or reintroducing it after having a fitness break or an operation... or a baby, of course. While I refer to mums throughout, and while the introduction deals with a lot of the physical changes that happen while pregnant or postpartum, please don't feel left out if that's not your situation. The pelvic floor exercises and core work are suitable for both women and men at any stage of life, the recipes are bloody delicious, whoever you are, and the self-care tips are universal.

THE BENEFITS YOU'LL SEE

- You'll feel more energetic and motivated.

- Your body will get stronger, leaner and more toned.

- You'll experience better quality of sleep (when you're allowed to sleep, that is).

- Your skin and eyes will become brighter and healthier.

- Your hair and nails will get stronger.

- You'll become more productive: taking the time to work out actually saves you time in the long run, because you have more energy and higher concentration levels.

- By strengthening your core and pelvic floor, you'll repair what's been stretched, pulled or even broken.

- By being kind to yourself and looking after your mental health, you'll build up resilience.

Of course there will be bad days when you feel like crap, because, hey, that's life. But you'll be in a better position to cope with those days if your all-round physical and mental health is stronger.

HOW THE BOOK WORKS

First up, I delve into my personal experiences of pregnancy and birth (WARNING: my birth story is not for the faint-hearted), and of being a new mum.

I hope my honesty about both the ups and the downs will strike a chord and make you feel less alone. I think talking about this kind of stuff – hormones, cellulite, social media pressure, having sex after having a baby, self-esteem, the size of your post-birth knickers (WTF?) – is integral when it comes to feeling less isolated and to recognising that you do have control over how you both feel and look going forwards.

After my personal story, you'll find the training plan, which is specially designed to strengthen the parts of your body that have been most tested during pregnancy, while giving birth and also postpartum. It's divided into three phases of four weeks each (so twelve weeks altogether) that will get tougher as you do. Please don't be intimidated by the words 'training plan' or 'fitness plan'. As I mentioned before, this is a very gentle introduction or reintroduction to fitness, taking into account the stresses and strains new mums' bodies will have gone through. It is not a get-fit-quick plan. Take it at your own pace and enjoy it! (Yes, I have total faith you will enjoy it eventually, once you begin to feel and see the difference.)

Next, you'll find seventy-five delicious recipes (pages 132–275) that you'll wonder how you ever survived without. There are breakfasts, snacks, lunches, dinners, desserts and drinks, all created with speed and nutrition in mind. They've been designed for busy people who want to fuel themselves and their families with tasty, nutritious and balanced meals. You should integrate these into your life during the training plan.

And last, but definitely not least, you'll find the wellbeing section, starting on page 276. All who enter here must shed any guilt for having 'me time', and must accept that self-care is essential. This section is packed with tips and strategies that have both calmed me down and built me up during the last couple of years.

So, are you ready for this? Then let's get cracking! (I genuinely couldn't think of a line there that didn't sound weird in a pregnancy and birth context: 'Let's dive in'? Absolutely not. 'Let's push on'? Unacceptable. Even 'cracking' is dubious, but I'm going with it.)

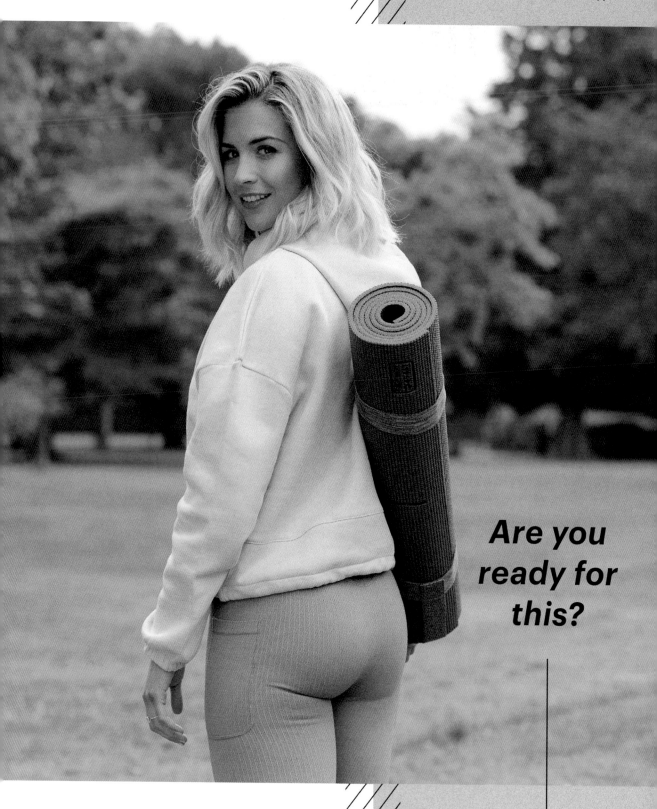

Are you ready for this?

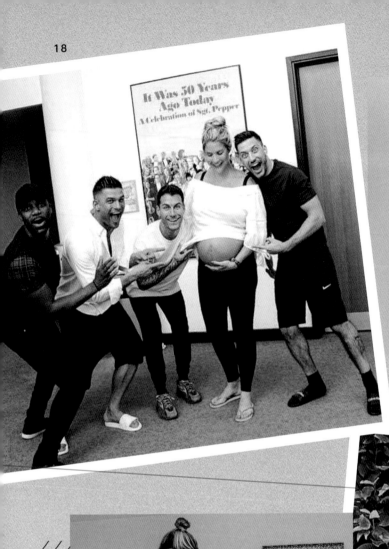

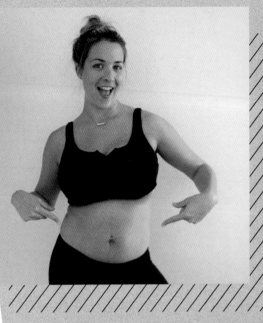

BUMPING ALONG NICELY

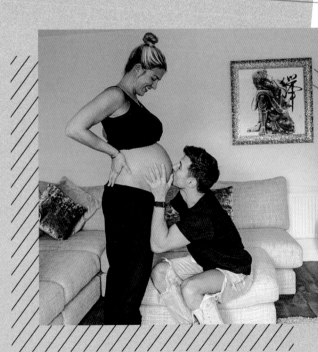

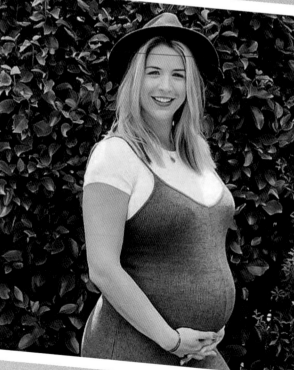

THE PREGNANCY TEST

For me, the whole experience of being pregnant can be summed up by one image: the exploding head emoji. It was joyful, nerve-wracking and all the emotions in between. It also made me feel both vulnerable and powerful – which sounds conflicting, because it is.

I'd never thought of myself as maternal before, because, if I'm totally honest, I never liked other people's children! I was always the person rolling my eyes at the screaming kid in the restaurant or scowling at the family sitting in the row behind me on the plane. Who doesn't love their chair being kicked by a screaming toddler for the duration of a four-hour flight? Of course, I adored my young relatives, but that's different, isn't it? The kids in your own family are always amazing, while everyone else's are monsters. It's funny though, because my mum always scoffed when I said I wasn't maternal, pointing out how my dogs are the most spoiled animals in the world (they do live like kings) and that my mates always come to me when they need a shoulder to cry on. I guess being 'maternal' is just about being loving to those you love.

While my elder sister, Nina, had always known she wanted kids and had three in her early twenties, motherhood really wasn't on my radar until Gorka and I discussed trying when we'd been together for just over a year. I'd known in a vague way that I'd like a family one day, but I had never felt in a position personally or professionally to consider it seriously. Then, at thirty-three years old, I was. I felt secure within my career, I'd travelled the world, I had my finances in place, I'd ticked a lot of things off my bucket list... and I was totally in love.

Gorka and I met while filming *Strictly Come Dancing* in 2017. He was one of the professional dancers and I was a contestant. And, even though we were both partnered with other people on the show, we started hanging out behind the scenes. After the main programme finished, the cast and crew spent two weeks touring the country together, and that was that: Gorka and I fell for each other. The whole team was crammed on the tour bus (more like the party bus) and Gorka and I got on ridiculously well – although I do remember thinking, 'I hope he's not this much of a party animal in real life!' Outside of *Strictly* and the tour, I had to get up at 4 a.m. every day for my radio show. There was no way I could party like this all the time – I'd die. Funnily enough, though, I later found out that Gorka was thinking exactly the same thing! Giovanni Pernice and Aljaž Škorjanec, two of the other professional *Strictly* dancers (Aljaž was my dance partner), said to me: 'We're so glad Gorka found you on this tour, because he was so boring on the last one – he'd be in bed by 9 p.m.!' When I heard that, I thought: 'Yes – my perfect match!'

I quickly realised I'd met someone very special. Gorka makes me feel beautiful even when I'm at my most disgusting. He makes me laugh until I wet myself. He looks after me and lets me look after him. He calls me out when I'm being an arse, and lets me call him out when he's being one. He's broken down my barriers, shown me a different side to myself, and supported me in everything I've wanted to do. He's the only boyfriend I've ever had that's made me think, 'Yes, let's make a mini-you or mini-me.' (Although we've both admitted that the thought of having to raise teenage versions of ourselves is terrifying!)

I look back at the relationships I was in during my mid-to-late twenties and think that if I'd had a baby with any of those people, I'd now be a single parent. Those relationships didn't work out for a reason. I'm still mates with some of my exes, as our break-ups were totally mutual, and some of the relationships were great at the time but definitely not long-term material. However, I've also experienced the other side: like many people, I've been cheated on and treated badly. You know, one guy took me on holiday even though, unbeknown to me, he had a girlfriend back home. He'd told her he was away with the lads! I mean, I laugh about it now, but WTF? Gorka was different – and I was different. Therefore, it felt like a no-brainer to come off the contraceptive pill in July 2018. What surprised us both, though, was that I became pregnant that October. I had no idea it would happen so quickly, and I know that makes us incredibly lucky. I have friends who have struggled to get pregnant or who have suffered miscarriages and I know my experience is not reflective of what many women go through. I felt incredibly grateful, but also very, very scared.

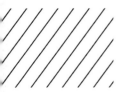

I quickly realised I'd met someone very special. Gorka makes me feel beautiful even when I'm at my most disgusting.

THE CLAPBACKS:
Tried-and-tested retorts to stupid comments

COMMENT:
'When are you having another?'
RESPONSE:
'When Gorka gets pregnant.'

COMMENT:
'You're just all bump, aren't you?'
RESPONSE:
'I know, it's like they call it a baby "bump" for a reason, right?'

COMMENT:
'You look like you're about to explode!'
RESPONSE:
'Cause I'm a firecracker, baby!'

COMMENT:
'You look shattered!'
RESPONSE:
'I'm not tired at all. You must be seeing things. Maybe you're the one who's tired?'

COMMENT:
'Are you going to breastfeed?'
RESPONSE:
'Why, do you want to try some milk?'

COMMENT:
'You're doing well walking round the park.'
RESPONSE:
'Got to keep fit for all that parasailing.'

COMMENT:
'Are you sure it's a girl? That's definitely a boy bump.'
RESPONSE:
'Thanks, I'll be sure to rely on your eyesight rather than the 4D scan I've just seen of my daughter's vagina.'

COMMENT:
'Was it an accident?'
RESPONSE:
'No, I definitely had sex on purpose.'

COMMENT:
'Are you sure you're only expecting one?'
RESPONSE:
'Yep. The rest is just bloating from all the beer I'm drinking.'

COMMENT:
'Enjoy this day trip/meal out/party while you can. You won't be doing it again for a while!'
RESPONSE:
'That means I probably won't bump into you for a while then, either, will I? Shame.'

COMMENT:
'Are you sure you should be doing/eating/ drinking/saying that?'
RESPONSE:
'Are you sure it's your business?'

COMMENT:
'Where's Mia?' (to me, despite Gorka standing right there too).
RESPONSE:
'Damn, babe! Did we leave her on the bus again?'

COMMENT:
'Can I touch your stomach?'
RESPONSE:
'Sure. I also have an itch on my lower back – could you give that a scratch, too?'

SCARY SECRETS

Obviously, everyone reacts differently to discovering they're pregnant, but for me it was like a giant flashing neon sign saying 'DANGER' had appeared over my head. I was suddenly very aware of my body and how seemingly fragile it was. An entirely new experience for me.

I was immediately worried about how my active lifestyle could potentially impact the baby. The fact that several of my friends had had problematic pregnancies and that much of the advice surrounding keeping the baby safe seemed to involve sitting motionless on the sofa for nine months really didn't help. I toned down my workouts dramatically – which was a big deal for me, as fitness is a huge part of my life – and found myself reticent to do things I normally wouldn't have thought twice about.

I remember during the first twelve weeks, I asked one of the guys at work to help me lift a box into my car. 'Come on! You can carry that!' he laughed. He meant it as a compliment, as I am usually proud of my strength and adamant that I can do things myself, but I had to make up some excuse about how I'd done my back in. The truth was, I was scared to lift the box in case I somehow hurt Mia. For the first time in my life, I felt physically vulnerable. I would whisper to my body: 'You can do those squats, and you can hike, and run for miles. Just look after my baby now, yeah? Please don't let me down.'

Before I had Mia, I was a total thrill-seeker. I'd thrown myself off the third-highest bungee jump in the world and swum with great white sharks. It was only ever afterwards that I'd think, 'Crikey, that could have gone either way, that.' I remember calling up my mum to tell her about the bungee jump and her screaming, 'YOU DID WHAT!?' down the phone so loudly it hurt my ears. She was absolutely fuming! Even more so when I then told her I had a DVD of the jump she could watch if she wanted! Now, though, I suddenly understood how she'd felt. It wasn't just my body to do whatever I liked with anymore. If I got hurt, Mia would suffer. That's a very weird thing to realise after feeling invincible your whole life. I was treating myself like I might break.

It doesn't help that, traditionally, you're not 'supposed' to tell people that you're expecting during the first trimester. I get it: if something goes wrong, you then have to tell them about that, too, and suffer the head tilts and pitying looks. But there's a lot to be said for the support you'll get. I'm so glad Gorka and I decided to tell our families and closest friends straight away. I would have gone mad if I hadn't. And, if something had gone wrong, I would have needed them. That doesn't mean I wanted to tell the whole world, though, which meant keeping the secret from the press. What was truly bizarre about that for me was that this secret showed on my body – and showing off my body was part of my job!

When I was about ten weeks pregnant, I was booked to do a fitness shoot. (It had been arranged before I knew I was pregnant.) I'd worked with the stylist a few times before, so she asked me if I was the same size as usual. I had to tell her: 'No, I'm two sizes bigger than I was last time we worked together.' I remember hearing the surprise in her reply. She must have been thinking: 'This fitness shoot has been booked in for months. What kind of lazy git doesn't train or prepare for it?' I'm there to promote staying consistent with your training, and yet am rocking up two sizes bigger without a word of explanation. I know some people don't show for ages, but I'd gone from training daily to doing nothing as I was afraid to, and my body had turned softer all over. The change in my body was more noticeable than it might be on lots of other people because I'd been so lean before. On top of that, I felt absolutely shocking on the day of the shoot, and couldn't squeeze my massive, swollen boobs into any of the sports bras they'd bought along. We had to get a new kit sent over, and the whole time I wanted to shout:

'I'M PREGNANT, OK? I'M TIRED AND BLOATED AND FEEL URGH.'

In another now-funny story, when I was two months pregnant, my friend Simon Rimmer, host of Channel 4's *Sunday Brunch*, asked me to be a guest on the show for an alcohol-tasting segment. He knew this would normally be a no-brainer for me, so was really confused when I said, 'Yes, I'll come on, but I don't drink anymore.'

'Okaaaay...' he replied. I'd just set fire to the entire point of the piece! It was awful hiding it.

So, when Gorka and I got the all-clear at the first scan, along with the huge relief of learning our baby was healthy, we also knew it was now 'safer' to start talking about the pregnancy publicly. We knew that didn't mean everything was automatically hunky-dory, but, rightly or wrongly, that twelve-week mark did act as a real boundary in my head. Finally, we could tell everyone! Hurray, right? Well... kind of. I'm going to admit something crazy here, but I found it really uncomfortable telling my older relatives I was pregnant, because it meant admitting that Gorka and I had had sex. Don't snort, I'm serious! I said to Gorka: 'Before, it might have been has-she, hasn't-she? They may have thought we had but they'd have never known.' But now they knew, officially, that we'd had sex – and without protection, no less! I told my best friend Laura how awkward I was finding it, and she said, 'Me too! I was so embarrassed telling my grandma. I wanted her to think it was an immaculate conception!' Gorka obviously thought I was completely mad, but come on: telling your Uncle Clive that you're pregnant is the same as saying, 'Hi Uncle Clive, guess what? Gorka and I had sex. Great, right?!' Don't tell me that's not *mortifying*.

Passing that milestone also made me feel more confident training again. As well as an adapted lightweight version of my usual workout routine, I took up Pilates, which I'd never done before, attending a class in Bury, which I loved. It was particularly good for me because my muscles get very tight from my usual workouts, so the stretching and elongating really helped me to feel less achy and sore. (We use a lot of yoga and Pilates-inspired exercises in the training plan in this book.) But, while very exciting, I also found it strange – and, yes, sometimes a bit scary – to see how quickly my body was changing as the pregnancy progressed.

THIS ROUTE HAS TOLLS

Pregnancy and having a baby exert a huge toll on the body. No matter what you do to prepare, or how fit or how zen you are, you will still sweat and swell up in places you didn't even know it was possible to sweat or swell up.

I gained enormous respect and appreciation for every woman who'd gone through this before. Never again will my eyes glaze over when a pregnant woman moans about carrying what feels like a bowling ball around 24/7. I FEEL YOU. And, on top of that, your hormones go completely mad. Your partner will become an expert at knowing when to gracefully exit an argument they're never going to win. You'll cry at nothing, laugh at nothing, be delighted at nothing and be devastated at nothing. All within the same five minutes. And that continues for a year, more or less.

Then there's the pregnancy police: people who think they get to tell you that whatever you're doing is wrong. 'You shouldn't eat that', 'You shouldn't drink that', 'Are you sure you should be doing that in your condition?' Here's a newsflash for people who think that it's a good idea to inform strangers on the internet about the dangers of pregnancy or provide them with 'helpful' tips: PREGNANT WOMEN KNOW THE RISKS. THEY ARE IN A PERPETUAL STATE OF ANXIETY. YOU DON'T HAVE TO MAKE IT WORSE. And strangers – people you've never met before in your entire life – will think they can touch your stomach: that, just because you're carrying a baby, it's somehow acceptable for them to stroke you. This really shouldn't need saying, but that's not OK. You can stroke my dogs if they like you, but not my belly!

And this police force doesn't go away after you've had a baby. Oh no! They were just warming up. Soon they graduate to the mum police: 'Why does your baby have a hat on when it's so hot?', 'Why doesn't your baby have a hat on when it's so cold?', 'Why is she in a sling when she's so young?', 'Why is she under a mosquito net when she may run out of oxygen?' (All comments I have personally experienced. Yes, even the mosquito net one.)

The last thing an expectant or new mum needs is judgement. You feel like you're doing everything wrong anyway. Mum guilt is real (see page 38), so trust in yourself, research for yourself and don't feel swayed by keyboard warriors (or, heaven forbid, people who stop you in the street!).

SEX, CELLULITE & SELF-ESTEEM

Once, when I was heavily pregnant and we were about to have sex, Gorka asked me, 'Do you think it might hurt the baby?'

I roared with laughter. 'Don't flatter yourself!' I lolled.

Having sex while up the duff is safe, normal and really good for your self-esteem. I think women put too much emphasis on the physical changes they've gone through, thinking, 'God, my partner won't fancy me while I'm huge and sweaty,' but it's not about fancying you at this stage (although they still will!) — it's about love, as cheesy as that sounds. All the partners I've spoken to confirm that sure, they may not be looking at their missus and thinking, 'Phwoar! Yeah!' at that moment, but they're actually feeling something much deeper and stronger: they're looking at the person carrying their baby. They all said that they loved their partner even more, seeing what they were going through — and these new stronger feelings included wanting to sleep with them. Don't hide away or fight the changes. You have to embrace them, and trust that your other half embraces them too.

I got really bad cellulite while pregnant, which may have been because of the oestrogen spike in my body (although there are lots of other things that can cause it). I mean, I have cellulite anyway, but this was next-level. Gorka said, 'You're pregnant, so what? That's normal.' He was right, but it can still be a shock to see a change like that on your own body. There's not much anyone can do about cellulite. A healthy lifestyle and diet will help, but hormones are hormones, and they go haywire during pregnancy. Getting upset and stressed about it is only going to make you feel worse. My dad always used to say: 'Worrying is like riding a rocking horse — it's something to do, but it'll get you nowhere.' So, after I had Mia, I drank loads of water, ate good food, started gently increasing my mobility and, as my hormones levelled off, the cellulite decreased. But it did affect my self-esteem. I also noticed that when you're massively pregnant, self-care can go out the window: it feels like a hassle to just move from one room to the next, let alone get a blow-dry. But don't neglect the things that make you feel better! One thing I did do was ask Gorka to shave my bikini line. I told him: 'You'll have to shave it for me, because I can't see it — and I'm not going to have the doctors and nurses thinking I'm unkempt.' I was nine months along and ready to pop and, bless him, he did it, and ended with a flourish, saying: 'It's a good job you can't see it, because I've done a diagonal mohawk!'

GIVING BIRTH:
Strap in for a bumpy ride

Mia was due on 22 July 2019 but was born on 4 July (an Independence Day baby!). To say her birth was not smooth sailing is as much of an understatement as saying Tom Hardy is alright looking.

Trigger warning: those with a nervous disposition should look away now and rejoin us on page 34. I am going to reveal details about emergency caesareans and haemorrhages that some people may find distressing, but what happened is an integral part of my motherhood journey and goes a long way towards explaining the toll that pregnancy and birth took on my body. Like a lot of new mums, I've had to negotiate a wealth of physical and mental repercussions since giving birth. It's not just a case of getting back to the gym or 'snapping back' (pfft!) when your body and your head aren't ready.

So – deep breath – here we go...

We'd planned for a water birth, but my mum had very firmly told me planning for anything was ridiculous, as babies do whatever they want. And boy, was she right. My waters broke on 2 July. I wasn't hugely worried about that happening nearly three weeks early, because I'd been practising hypnobirthing, which is all about using breathing techniques, mindfulness and visualisation to stay relaxed and help manage the pain. My fabulous hypnobirthing teacher had told me, 'Don't focus on a specific date, just say your baby's coming in July. Women put themselves under so much pressure thinking they're either early or late, when in reality, the baby will come when the baby is ready.'

But apparently Mia wasn't ready to come. I spent the rest of that day and evening at home, bouncing on a ball, lying in the garden, pacing up and down... and nothing. The next morning (3 July) the midwife told us to go to the hospital and they'd try to get things going to minimise the risk of infection. So my mum, Gorka and I headed off. But again, nothing happened. We spent the whole of that day waiting, but nada. Zilch. Bupkis. Mia was having none of it.

The thing that makes me laugh now, knowing how it panned out, is that on 4 July, the day everything kicked off, Gorka was sitting there watching Wimbledon on his laptop. He had the Nadal game on (FYI, it was the second round and Nadal beat Kyrgios in four sets) and he was 'ooohing' and 'aahing' at every point. I didn't mind because there was nothing else to do! By this stage, I'd supposedly been in labour for thirty-six hours, but still hadn't had a single contraction. I'd been given a pen-like device attached to a machine and was told to click it each time I felt Mia kick. Eventually, a nurse came in, checked the clicking and, concern flashing across her face, told me I'd be given

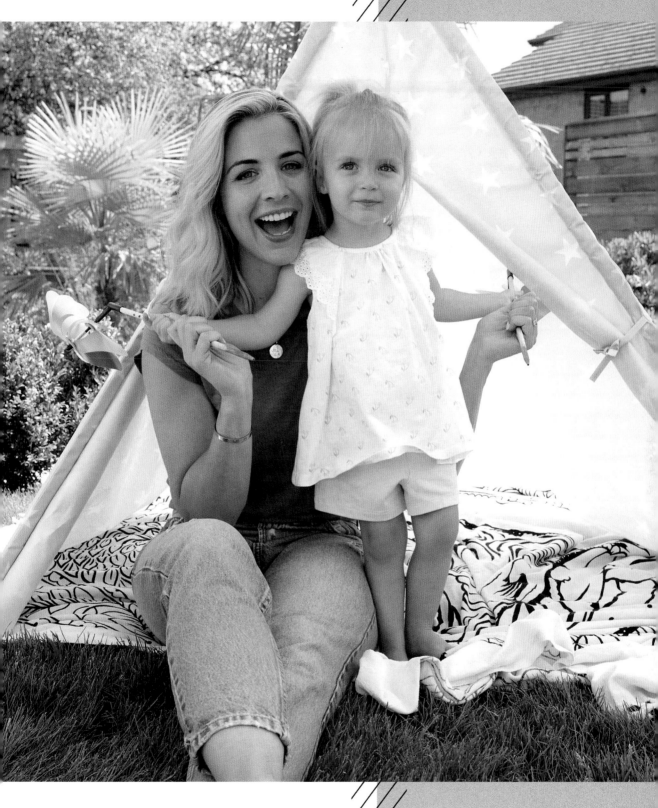

The Ultimate Body Plan for New Mums

a 'sweep'. This is when they sweep their fingers around your cervix to try to trigger labour. But Mia was still unimpressed, determined to stay in my belly. It was probably all her dad's 'ooohing' at Nadal that made her think, 'Sack that – I'm staying in here!'

By mid-afternoon, they announced that they were going to induce me. They figured Mia was simply too small to push herself out, especially since my muscles were so tight from years of training. (This was the first time I'd heard anyone say that she was small. During all of our scans, we'd been told she was a big, healthy baby). I was warned that, once I'd been induced, the contractions would start very quickly and be very painful – and they weren't lying. The first contraction reminded me of being kicked in the stomach when I'd done Muay Thai boxing once. But hey – at least things were moving now, right?

Wrong!

I was looking at the doctor's face as she watched Mia's heart rate on the screen, and I saw at once that things weren't OK. She leaned over, took my hand and softly said, 'Mia's heartbeat should be between one hundred and ten and one hundred and sixty, and it's dropped to forty. We have to get her out right now. I'm going to press a button that will sound an alarm, and lots of people are going to come in. Don't panic. Stay calm. Whatever happens, you're going to meet your baby today.'

Then she hit the alarm: BEEP BEEP BEEP! And suddenly the room was full of people in scrubs shouting at each other. They started wheeling me out and, stunned, I looked over at my mum, who smiled and gave me the thumbs up. Gorka later told me that as soon as I left, she burst into tears. He couldn't comfort her, though, because the doctor told him to hurry up and get his scrubs on. My poor mum was left alone, wondering what on earth was going on, and what was happening to *her* baby – bless her.

They took me into theatre and administered the epidural at about 4 p.m. People had told me how painful the injection was, but I didn't find that at all. In fact, I didn't even know I'd had it until I noticed I'd lost control of my bladder and had wet myself. 'I'm so sorry,' I whimpered. 'I've just been to the toilet!' One of the doctors or nurses said, 'Don't worry, lovey, that's the least of our worries,' and cleaned me up without batting an eyelid. I lay down and a doctor prodded my belly, asking if I could feel it. I said yes. They all looked at each other.

'If this epidural doesn't kick in soon,' one of them explained, 'we're going to have to put you to sleep, because we need to get this baby out now.'

And that's when I panicked. Up until then, I'd been convinced that everything would be OK. But this wasn't OK, because not only did I desperately want to be awake when Mia arrived, but I also knew that if I was put under, Gorka wouldn't be allowed in the room.

'Please, please – just wait a bit longer!' I sobbed.

The doctor sprayed something ice cold on my stomach and I flinched.

'You felt that, didn't you, Gemma?' she asked.

'No, I didn't!' I lied. When I saw they hadn't bought it, I said, 'Just do it anyway! I'll be fine!' I was really crying now, and the doctors were all talking over each other, trying to decide what to do. What would take longer: fully knocking me out, or waiting for the epidural to work? What was the bigger risk?

At that moment, Gorka burst in wearing these *enormous* scrubs. They were hanging off him. I remember saying to him, through my tears, 'They're too big for you, they are.'

He said, 'I know – look!' He stuck out his arms and legs in a star shape, and the sleeves flopped over his hands. I laughed – actually laughed – and then the nurse was saying, 'OK, we're good to go now. The epidural has kicked in.'

The op started, and I was pushed and pulled about a bit because they were rushing so much, but the next thing I knew, they were holding Mia up in the air, like Simba in *The Lion King*. My gunky, bloody, beautiful, tiny little lion. She started crying and I thought, 'Thank God she's here.'

Bloody terrifying

There followed a couple of hours of loveliness. It's true the birth hadn't gone to plan (if you listen hard, you'll still be able to hear my mum saying, 'I told you so'). I mean, Gorka hadn't even been able to cut the umbilical cord, for goodness' sake. ('This is much harder than it looks,' he'd muttered.) But Mia was out – healthy and beautiful and all ours! We were taken to a recovery ward, where she was weighed, we officially recorded her name, and Mum and Peter, my stepdad, got to meet her. After we'd taken 20,000 photos, they said goodbye and headed home, swinging by Asda on their way to pick up some miniature baby clothes because at only 4lb 10oz, everything we'd bought for Mia swamped her. She looked like a little rat, bless her.

So there I was, chatting to Gorka, Mia lying peacefully in the cot next to me, when suddenly it was like someone had flipped a switch. I felt simply *awful*. It was unlike anything I've ever experienced before, and I knew something was really wrong. Gorka said all the colour drained from my face, and I looked as white as a ghost. I felt a mixture of light-headed, bone-tired and travel sick. 'I think you need to get somebody,' I whispered, and he ran to fetch a nurse. She stepped inside our privacy curtain, whipped my blanket back and we all stared. The entire bed was sodden with dark red blood, which was flowing from between my legs. I hadn't felt a thing, because I was still numb from the epidural.

The next thing I knew, they were holding Mia up, like Simba in **The Lion King.** *My gunky, bloody, beautiful, tiny little lion.*

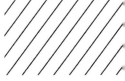

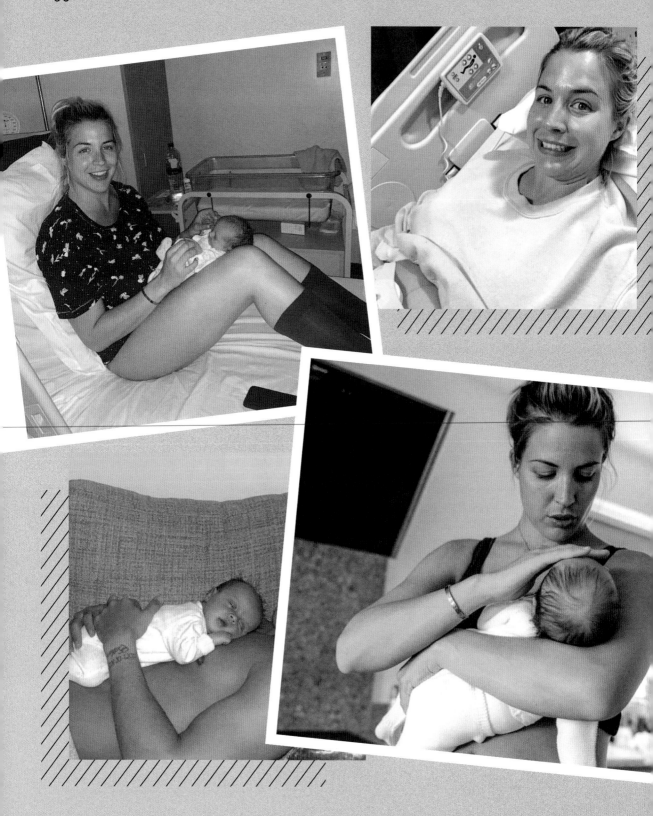

For the second time in only a couple of hours, someone hit the panic button and all hell broke loose. Gorka later described it as like a Formula One pit stop – all these doctors running in, flapping around the bed, connecting me to IVs, taking my vitals. It was equal parts amazing and terrifying. I was thinking, 'Wow! Look at how efficient they are!' and then, 'Wait – if the professionals are freaking out, how bad must it be?' It was particularly scary for Gorka, who's Spanish. English is his second language. In fact, it's actually more like his third language, after Portuguese. He was desperately trying to understand what was happening; what all the shouting was about.

I can still picture the face of the young doctor who was trying to keep me calm. He was wonderful. He was looking into my eyes and asking, 'What's your baby called? Tell me your baby's name.' I was saying, 'Mia! She's called Mia! Where is she? Is she OK? Can you get her for me? What's happened to her?' And then, bizarrely, I turned and started shouting at Gorka: 'Don't let them take Mia!'

It sounds insane now, but all I could think was that if I died, they would take her away, and he might get a different baby back! Can you credit it?! I mean, I was well and truly out of it on all the pain meds, but my maternal instincts had kicked in. This was my first experience of how my priorities had changed: I had this overwhelming fear that something would happen to her if I died. Because, yes, I did think I might die. I'm not even sure why, but I remember clearly thinking: 'Right. If this is it, this is it. I'm going to die in this hospital and my daughter isn't going to know me... but I'll see my dad again soon and he'll make it all OK.' (My dad died when I was 17.) I can't explain how shocking it is to see a pint of blood spreading across a bed – your blood. I don't subscribe to any religion, but I do believe there's something out there, something bigger than us, and I found it peaceful to think I'd see my dad again. I just wanted Mia to know how much I'd wanted her... and to make sure Gorka got to keep the right baby (don't ask).

So, there's this doctor trying his best to calm me down, me thinking I'm going to die, a nurse massaging my tummy, another pulling jelly-like clots out of me, and yet another injecting me with something. I looked around for Gorka and saw him sitting in the corner on a chair, with his head between his legs, a nurse rubbing his back, telling him to take deep breaths. He'd nearly fainted! All these doctors and nurses are trying to stop me bleeding, and he was there getting on the gas and air! The whole scene was ridiculous, like a *Carry On* film. I can only apologise to the other women in the ward, who had to listen to all this and must have been clutching their newborns in absolute horror. But then, whatever medication they'd put me on, or whatever it was they'd done must have started working, because someone said: 'She won't need a blood transfusion.' I thought, 'Grand,' then, 'Wait – what?! I might have needed a blood transfusion?'

When the danger was over, they took me to another room (I'd seen a lot of recovery rooms by this point) to clean up the mess. In the lift, I asked: 'Is this normal? Does this happen to lots of people? Am I going to be OK?'

The nurse said, 'Don't worry, Gemma. You're fine. It's all over now.'

Only then did I allow my body to relax and I fell asleep.

'Will you stop having these episodes, Gemma?'

In total, I spent seven days in hospital. Two waiting to have Mia, and five recovering from the haemorrhage.

It's normal to bleed after giving birth. Blood naturally seeps from where the placenta was attached, and also from any tears or cuts that have occurred during labour. This 'normal' bleeding is heaviest just after birth and reduces over the next few days, the blood turning from red to brown. It's called lochia and should have stopped altogether by the time your baby is six weeks old.

Obviously, that's not what happened to me. I had what's called a postpartum haemorrhage (PPH). 'Primary PPH' (what I had) is when you lose more than 500ml of blood within the first twenty-four hours after birth. Depending on when and where it happens (i.e. if you're in the hospital or at home), and what your physical condition is when it kicks off, it shouldn't be life-threatening but will still be taken seriously by the medical staff looking after you. Most women will have a 'minor' haemorrhage, which is when you lose between 500ml and 1000ml of blood (1–2 pints). A 'severe' haemorrhage (when you lose more than 1 litre or 2 pints of blood) is much less common. This often requires more treatment such as a blood transfusion, and medicine or a procedure to stop the bleeding. It's worth noting that if you have a PPH, you might become anaemic and tired, and it can take a few weeks before you make a full recovery. A secondary PPH is when you have heavy vaginal bleeding between twenty-four hours and twelve weeks after the birth. It can be a sign of infection or some placenta still in the womb – but this is also really rare. Although it doesn't sound like it, I was actually very lucky. The fact I was in the hospital when it started meant I had the best possible care, and I'd like to thank everyone at Bolton Royal for their professionalism and kindness from start to finish.

It's funny what you remember after a crisis. I have a couple of super-vivid images in my head from that time. When I was in the recovery room feeling incredibly sick, the midwife, Diane, immediately grabbed one of those cardboard bowls that are everywhere in hospitals and held it under my mouth. As I was throwing up, I just kept watching my vomit rise and rise in the bowl, and all I could think was, 'It's going to touch her thumb!' I was mortified. And then there was the moment my mum and Peter burst in, having legged it back from buying the baby clothes in Asda. Gorka had called to tell them about the haemorrhage, and my mum told me they'd sprinted across Asda's carpark carrying this bag of clothes, looking like they'd just nicked them and were doing a runner. As she hugged me, she asked: 'Have you finished now, Gemma? Will you stop having these episodes?' I replied that I hoped so.

A week or so after it happened, I started having terrible nightmares. Gorka was away on tour, and my mum had moved in to help with Mia as there wasn't much I could do with my stitches. She had to come into my room several times to comfort me as I screamed out in my sleep. You know how, during a big night out, you don't really process what's happening moment by moment? And it's only during the following days you start remembering the details? It was like that. I'd have moments that I'd suddenly think, 'Woah! What if that had gone differently?' and feel overwhelmed. It got to a point when every time I went to sleep, I would say, 'Please let me wake up in the morning.' I'd never felt like that before. I even rang the doctor and asked him to change my medication, because I was on some heavy-duty painkillers that made me feel even more on edge.

I also wondered what I'd done wrong. Did I eat the wrong things when I was pregnant? Did I train too hard? Could it have been those antibiotics I took for that water infection? I think it's in our nature to blame ourselves. Telling myself it was my fault gave me a sense of control over a situation that felt very out of control. If I could blame it on X, Y or Z, I thought, then, if we had another baby, I'd be able to stop it happening again.

I've always said I want Mia to have a sibling because I'm so close to my older sister, Nina, and Gorka is close to his brother, Jonathan. But for a long time after the birth, I said to Gorka: 'I can't go through that again. Nope. No way. I'd be scared to death my whole pregnancy.' Men like to say, 'A kick in the bollocks is more painful than having a baby.' They definitely don't turn around a year later and say, 'Hey, do you fancy kicking me in the bollocks again?' Yet women say, 'Shall we have another baby?' I won't ever forget what I went through (see page 26), but now I know I absolutely would go through it all again in a heartbeat, because I'd love for Mia to have a little brother or sister. So, yes, we'll try again – as soon as Mia can tie her own laces and wipe her own bum.

Staff at the hospital told me that if I ever wanted to know exactly what happened and why, they'd sit down and talk it through with me – and at first, I really thought I'd take them up on the offer. An emergency caesarean and then a haemorrhage – it was by no means an ideal birth story. But after a while, I changed my mind. I don't want to dwell on it. I can't change it, and I want to move on.

Someone said to me once, 'I've heard Mia's birth wasn't great.'

My mum piped up and said, 'Oh no! Mia had a successful birth – a really successful birth!'

I just stared at her.

'Well,' she said, 'you're here and Mia's here, so it's a success! No matter how you got through it, at the end of the day, you want a healthy baby and a healthy mum, and that's what you got.'

OK, Mum. You can have that one.

I thought, 'You know what? She's right.' Yes, Mia was tiny, and the odds were stacked against her, but she made it! She came out fighting – and on Independence Day, of all days! This was Mia's way of coming into the world; she wanted to make an entrance. And besides, how bad was it really? Gorka even got to watch a bit of Wimbledon!

MIA, MYSELF AND I

One minute you're pregnant, and the next you're holding a baby thinking, 'WTF just happened?' I don't know if everyone reading this will be like, 'Well, what did you expect?' but for me, I felt pretty shell-shocked returning home.

It was like I should somehow magically know exactly what to do and how to feel – and I didn't. There was this feeling that all other parents just automatically know what they're doing, but I'd somehow missed the memo. I remember I had to ask my mum to help me bathe Mia, because I'd never bathed a baby before.

On top of all that, your body feels like it belongs to a stranger. Whether you had a vaginal birth or a caesarean, your body is traumatised, and you feel, to put it bluntly, revolting.

One of the funniest examples of this was when the health visitor came round to check in, a couple of days after we'd got back from the hospital. I hadn't had a poo in days. Lots of people had warned me that the first post-birth poo would be difficult, but I'd never expected this. I was so constipated, it was unbearable. So there I was, sitting on the loo with a poo half out of my bottom when the doorbell rang. I heard my mum welcome the health visitor and say, 'Gem's just in the toilet. She won't be long.' I just thought, 'OH MY GOD.' I couldn't move and nothing was happening down there at all. I was rocking backwards and forwards with sweat pouring down my face, and I could hear them making small talk. I thought I was going to pass out. I must have been in there for twenty minutes. When I finally staggered into the living room, sweating and panting, there was this silence. Later, when my mum and I were waving the health visitor off, she said to me out of the corner of her mouth: 'Bet you need some Sudocrem on your arse, don't you?' We both cracked up, laughing so hard we couldn't stop. Howling and crying in the hallway. And wow, I really needed that laugh! It felt like a bit of normality. Like everything was going to be OK.

Another disgusting thing (sorry, I'm on a roll), was when I got mastitis. Mastitis is when your boobs become hot, swollen and painful from breastfeeding. It hurts like hell. The only relief I found was a remedy suggested by my mum: frozen cabbage leaves on my nipples. The blessed relief of those leaves! Beautiful! The trouble is though, you put the frozen leaves down your bra... and then they defrost and smell like farts. I'd forget they were in there, sit down on the sofa and – ooof! This awful smell would woosh up my nose, and I'd be looking round to see who'd farted – and then realise it was my boobs! And I figured: sod snapping back – this is the stuff people should be talking about!

10 THINGS NO ONE TELLS YOU WILL HAPPEN AFTER HAVING A BABY

1/ You'll have to wear Bridget Jones-style massive knickers to fit the industrial-sized sanitary pads you need. (*And then you'll never want to wear any other kind, because these enormous pants are so goddamn comfy. Thongs? Yeah, right. Lol.*)

2/ All the lovely cosmetics and lotions in your cupboards will be replaced by Sudocrem. And haemorrhoid cream.

3/ Having a poo is a seriously stressful event. (*Please refer back to no. 2.*)

4/ Wanting to have sex? Hahahaha.

5/ You will never 'pop out' anywhere ever again. Every attempt to leave the house will become a military operation. I got to sub-ten minutes during Month Four, but then realised I'd forgotten Mia's wipes. Dammit!

6/ You'll laugh at your past self for ever thinking you were tired.

7/ At some point, you will definitely cry over spilt milk. (*I broke during week five at 3 a.m.*)

8/ Dry shampoo will become your new best friend.

9/ The joy of having had no periods for nine months will be swiftly obliterated by the bloody madness you'll experience the first few weeks after giving birth. Expect anything from spotting to a full-on murder scene in your sanitary pad.

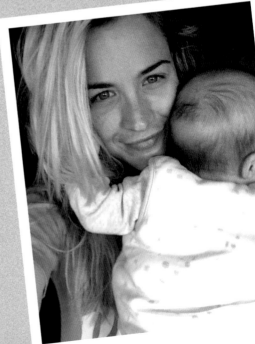

10/ Daytime TV becomes your saviour. I couldn't wait for *A Place in the Sun* and *Dickinson's Real Deal*.

A labour of love

Another thing people don't talk about enough is the jealousy you'll feel of your partner and of your past life. Gorka had to go away on tour pretty soon after Mia's birth, and I remember seeing pictures of him and the boys in the gym or mucking about. I called him in tears, saying, 'I can't do any of that. I can't exercise, go see my friends, go to work. I can't even wash my own hair.' I suddenly couldn't do a lot of what made me 'me', or the things I'd always done to keep me feeling good. Then, two weeks later, Gorka called me up in tears, saying all he wanted to do was to be at home with us. 'It's OK for you,' he said. 'You're at home with our little girl, while I'm on the road, away from both of you.' It made us realise we were both craving a bit of what the other had. I'm so glad we spoke about it and realised what the other was going through. It definitely brought us closer together and gave us both a different perspective on things.

And speaking of perspectives, it certainly gave us an entirely new view of sex. Safe to say, slipping into some Agent Provocateur undies and slinking into the bedroom was about as far from my mind as attempting another bungee jump. I think it was a good seven or eight weeks after Mia was born that we even gave it a go, and that first time was just plain awkward. So awkward, in fact, it was hilarious.

'Where can I go?'

'Not there, because of my stitches. Can you put a pillow under here?'

'How about there?'

'Ouch! No, that won't work either. Is it weird that Mia's in the room? What if she sees?'

'Gemma, she's less than two months old.'

And then, when we finally got into a comfortable position, my breasts started leaking milk! It was the least sexy thing in the entire world – so much so, we ended up laughing our heads off about it. After that, things could only get better, to be fair.

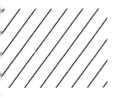

I suddenly couldn't do a lot of what made me 'me', or the things I'd always done to keep me feeling good.

WHY YOU MAY FEEL SAD,
MAD OR JUST PLAIN BAD

Your hormones lose their tiny minds while you're pregnant – and they don't immediately get their shit together the moment you give birth. Without getting too bogged down in the science, let's just say your body is flooded with hormones while you're up the duff – and then the levels drop off dramatically after the baby arrives. They're like: 'Job done! Cheers, lads. We're off!', leaving you feeling off-kilter, to say the least.

You may hear people refer to the 'baby blues'. It's an incredibly patronising term that nevertheless should reassure you that feeling down after having a baby is common. The 'baby blues' usually disappear within one to two weeks. However, postnatal depression is a very different beast and recognising the symptoms so you can differentiate between the two is very important:

- **BABY BLUES:** feeling a bit down, tearful or anxious in the first week or two after giving birth.

- **POSTNATAL DEPRESSION:** not just feeling a bit down, but sad to the point of hopelessness. You might also be anxious, fatigued and disinterested in everything – even the stuff that used to give you pleasure (and even your new baby). You may suffer from frightening thoughts of harming yourself or others, and feel guilty about pretty much everything, blaming yourself for feeling that way. These feelings will last for weeks or months.

There is also prenatal depression, which is much less widely known, but just as important. This is when you experience the same symptoms as postnatal depression, but during pregnancy.

If feelings of sadness persist for longer than two weeks (either prenatal or post) and you recognise several of the symptoms listed above, please speak to your health worker or GP. And, most importantly, don't blame yourself: depression is an illness, not a flaw. Please seek help – it can be treated.

LOOKING AFTER YOURSELF IS NOT SELFISH

You may feel as if taking some time out each day to train or practise the self-care tips in the wellbeing section is in some way selfish. It's absolutely not. Looking after yourself is the most unselfish thing you could do for the good of your family.

You should not feel guilty about it – nor should you push yourself too hard. Remember to listen to your body. Go at your own pace and be kind to yourself.

Mum guilt is real, and I have no magic formula to stop it. I feel guilty when Mia is at my sister's while I'm at work; when Gorka and I have a date night; or when she's at my mum's and Peter's for a playdate. All totally natural, normal and healthy things for all of us to be doing, yet I'll feel guilty about it. I even felt guilty about my mum staying with me after the birth, thinking, 'She's in her sixties, she should be chilling out, not washing my hair for me.' But when I asked her if she minded, she snorted. 'This is my job as your mum,' she said. 'Your nana did it for me, and you'll do it for Mia one day, too – and you'll love it.'

My message is this: it's not selfish to look after yourself, or to want to better yourself, and you're already doing so much better than you think you are! Just by picking up this book, you're making a commitment to change how you feel about yourself, and that's something to be encouraged and celebrated. This is a journey that will change your life – and I'm so proud you're taking it with me.

Start taking photographic evidence of your awesomeness

When I was packing up my house to move in September 2020, I found lots of old family photos in the loft – including many of my dad. I can't explain how grateful I was to come across these pictures. Not only because they reminded me of times we'd shared together, but also because one day, I'll be able to show the pictures to Mia.

It made me realise how sad it is that so many people don't take pictures of themselves. People post lots of snaps of their kids online, but rarely appear in the pics with them. When scrolling through friends' albums, I sometimes ask, 'Wait, where were you?' and they'll say, 'Oh, I looked shocking that day!' or 'No, no one wants to see me.' But that's so untrue. Your kids want to see you. Your friends and family want to see you. And, believe

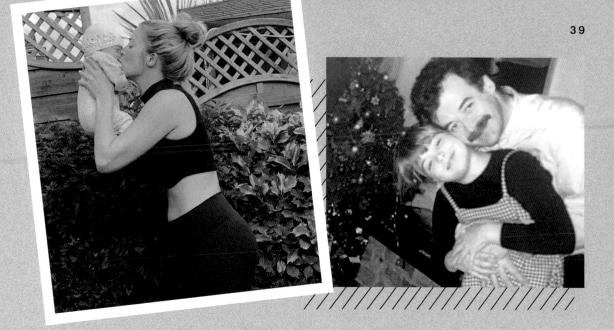

it or not, one day, you will want to see yourself. I am so thankful for every photo I have of my dad, whether they are ones with me in, too, or just snaps of him going about his business. It's a record of a moment we'll never have again, but that I can treasure forever. Social media has changed how we view taking photos and videos. They're no longer just for personal albums or to stick on the fridge – they're for hundreds of people to rate with a thumbs up or a heart. But I want to help change that mindset. I would love for readers of this book to start taking photos of themselves – for themselves and their family (social media is optional!). That's why I've recommended it as one of the ways in which you'll track your progress during this plan (see page 70).

It's not just about you anymore. If you avoid cameras and tell people you don't look good enough to be in a photo, what message is that passing on to your kids? You're not only depriving them of keepsakes, but also saying that only certain ways of looking are good enough to be recorded. Trust me, you're not going to regret appearing in a photo having a laugh with your family – but you will regret not appearing in any. We've got a picture of Mia and me that is hilariously bad. She's about a month old and I'm lying with her on the floor. My belly's out, and I'm just wearing knickers and a huge postpartum sanitary pad. Gorka took the pic and showed me. 'Bloody hell!' I gasped. 'Look at the state of me in that!' I even sent it to my girlfriends, with the caption: 'Here's one of FHM's 100 Sexiest Women in the World!' But really – who cares if I look like total shite? The point is Mia's in my arms, and I'm absolutely delighted. I went through hell to get her, and one day she'll look at that photo and know how wanted she was.

Training and eating well will help with your confidence appearing in photos – not just because you'll *look* fitter, but also because you'll *feel* better about yourself. You'll realise your body is amazing, whatever size or shape you are, and having a record of these moments is more important than trying to measure up to any idealised version of 'perfect'.

5 NEW-MUM MYTHS BUSTED

1/ I'LL MAGICALLY FORGET ALL ABOUT THE BIRTH

As should be clear from the introduction, I haven't forgotten Mia's birth – and I don't think I ever will. Some women have to have trauma counselling after what they've been through, and minimising that by adhering to a belief that you should magically forget all about it isn't healthy. Women are not biologically 'programmed' to forget childbirth. How much you remember and what you remember depends on lots of factors, including: whether the birth went 'to plan'; whether any medical intervention was necessary; what level of care you received and how satisfied you were with it; where you were and who you were with; how much pain you experienced; and the outcome for your baby. We may also retrospectively play down what happened as a coping mechanism. What you remember and how much you remember is entirely personal, so please don't think there's something wrong with you if the memories remain vivid – and do seek counselling if you think talking about it will help.

2. I'LL NEVER SETTLE INTO A 'NEW NORMAL'

OK, so life will never be the same again. That's a given. But you will settle into your new normal, I promise. Things won't always feel this huge. It would be weird to slide seamlessly into a new life without batting an eyelid. Any monumental change takes getting used to, so take things one day at a time. Practising simple self-care tips (see page 282) can make the world of difference when it comes to how manageable things feel, and it will remind you that you're still *you* – you're just experiencing a brand-new side to yourself.

3. I MUST ENJOY EVERY SINGLE MOMENT

People will have probably said to you at some point: 'Enjoy every minute! It goes by so fast!' This is one of those off-the-cuff comments that seems harmless, but if you hear it often enough, you might start to wonder if you're wrong for sometimes feeling shattered or shell-shocked by the madness of your new life. Constantly feeling like dancing for joy when you're covered in sick is simply not realistic, so don't feel guilty or like a bad mum during your down times. You don't need any additional pressure right now, so ditch the self-judgement. Allow yourself moments of ugh, meh and bleurgh – accept them as normal and natural. It'll make the genuinely great moments even better.

4. EVERYONE ELSE KNOWS WHAT THEY'RE DOING

No one knows what they're doing! Everyone is blagging it. Yes, even Perfect Polly with her just-the-right-side-of-cute matching mum-and-daughter outfits on Facebook. Trust your instincts. Someone said to me once: 'You'll know when Mia's crying and you'll know when she's really *crying*.' I was like, 'What do you mean? What if I don't know?' But they were right – now I know! Mia has a fake cry, a tired cry and a real cry. I can be on the phone and she'll be standing in front of me, fake-crying, and the person on the other end will go, 'Oh! Do you need to see to Mia?' And I'll say, 'No, she's right in front of me, pretending to cry.' But then other times, there's the real cry – when she's scared or in pain – and it takes my breath away. That's instinct. Trust it. And when you don't know what to do, ask someone you trust who does! I've asked my mum for advice non-stop: whether Mia should have two blankets at night or a sleep suit; whether she was big enough to start weaning; even whether it was normal for her poo to have a seed-like appearance despite her not having eaten seeds! (FYI, it's completely normal for a breastfed baby to have seedy poop.) After all, my mum raised me and I think I turned out OK!

5. YOU'LL NEVER HAVE ALONE TIME OR 'COUPLE TIME' AGAIN

I hated being told this! I was also constantly told to kiss goodbye to my sex life and relationship, because 'once a baby comes, that all goes out the window'. Now, don't get me wrong, for the first two months after Mia's birth, sex was the last thing on my mind. Christ, I couldn't even see my vagina (due to my C-section bandages) – I didn't want Gorka anywhere near it. Over time, though, when I started to get into my routine, things started to get back to 'our normal'. I think it actually did me good to start feeling sexy again – and what better way to do that than have your partner make love to you or cuddle you or hold your hand on a stroll? Even just curling up together on the sofa to watch a film (during which you'll probably fall asleep because you're so tired) is still doing something together. One of my best friends is a single parent, and she said she bought herself some nice underwear and slapped on some body lotion, and it did her the world of good. She'd actually forgotten how hot she looked in a matching bra and pants, and she sent us all the pic on our group WhatsApp! Some couples do a date night once a week, some once a month. Some even book 'alone time' in separate rooms for a night. Whatever works for you and your family is right, so do what you need to do to keep things fresh and to feel your sexy-ass self again.

Allow yourself moments of ugh, meh and bleurgh – accept them as normal and natural. It'll make genuinely great moments even better.

THE FUTURE'S BRIGHT...

By following this plan, you can feel like *you* again. You can feel stronger, healthier, calmer and much more confident. The fact that you've picked up this book means you're up for making changes. That's a huge deal. The next step is making the choice to give this plan your all, come what may. Yes, it will involve making sacrifices and being stern with yourself – but if you really try, I promise that it will change your life. Eating well, training effectively and looking after myself has made me who I am today – a proud mother, sister, aunt and friend. And you're not just doing it for yourself or the here and now, you're doing it for your new family and for the future.

My grandad (my mum's dad) was an amazing man, but whenever I think of him in his later life, it's as a silent figure in his wheelchair. He smoked a lot and eventually had a stroke (we were told his smoking was a contributing factor for the stroke) and after this he lost his ability to speak. He was really active and playful with my sister and I when we were young, but he couldn't play with my sister's children at all. He'd just sit and smile at us so we knew he was OK, but Nina's kids missed out on knowing their great-grandad at his best. When I look at Mia now with my stepdad Peter, he's on his hands and knees playing with her or throwing her up in the air, and she's having the time of her life. She's going to remember her grandad as this lively presence, someone full of fun who would roll about on the floor with her. That's the quality of life I want for myself as I get older. I want to be throwing my own grandkids in the air. Sure, some things are out of our control – no one knows what's around the corner – but there are aspects of healthy living you *can* control. You can at least give yourself the best chance of being able to go hiking with your grandkids (or even great-grandkids!).

I'm so proud that you're going to take this journey with me towards becoming a healthier, happier you. You're not just a mum – you're also a badass friend, sibling, daughter, colleague, partner, neighbour and aunt, who's committed to finding themselves again! Welcome to *The Ultimate Body Plan for New Mums*! Let's go!

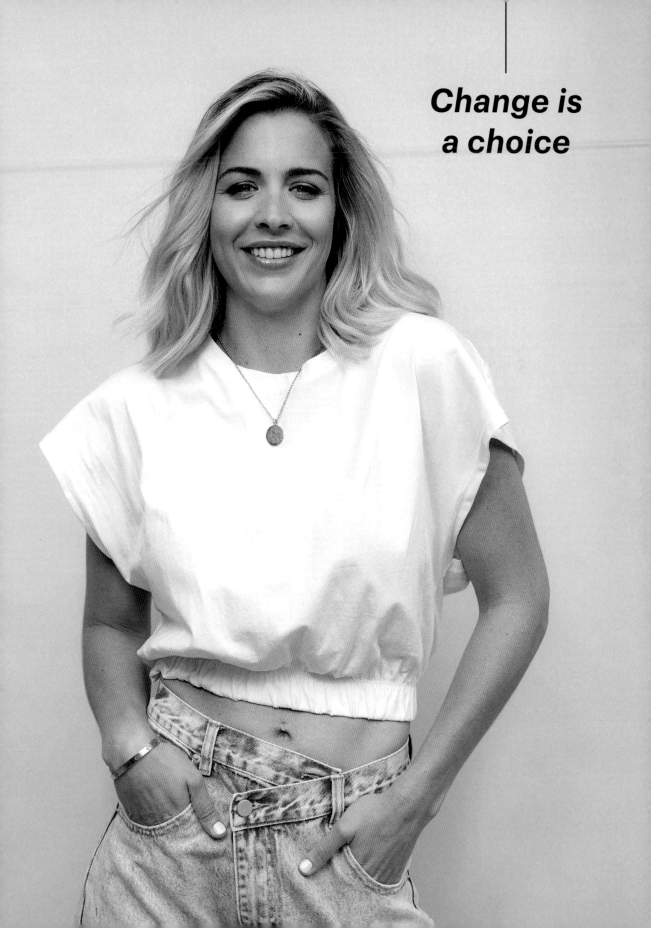

Change is
a choice

MY TEN COMMANDMENTS FOR FINDING 'YOU' AGAIN

These are the ten commandments you should follow during this twelve-week plan. They are empowering mantras, reminders and missives that will get you to where you want to be.

To succeed, you have to make yourself accountable for your own health and wellbeing. You must commit to wanting to feel better, healthier and stronger. See this as a vow to yourself that you're taking the plan seriously and won't jack it in as soon as things get tough. These commandments will provide reassurance and boost your resilience. They're about self-belief and self-worth. If it helps, make your favourite commandments into phone alerts that ping up at random times during the day, or write them on sticky notes and leave them around your house. They're there to remind you why you're doing this and of everything you have to gain.

1/ I WILL REMEMBER THAT I WAS SOMEONE BEFORE I WAS A MUM

Before I was a mother, I was a businesswoman, friend, daughter, sister, actor, presenter, adventurer, aunt... The list goes on. And I am still all of those things! I've just added 'mum' to the list. Motherhood doesn't define me, and that's OK, because I want Mia to be raised by well-rounded parents with lots of interests. I want her to be inspired by my career, friends and family. I want her to know that I have a past, present and future – a future that I am proud to invest in by working through this plan and looking after myself. I can switch from 'mum mode' to 'training mode' to 'gin-and-tonics-with-the-girls mode', and that's great. So remember: you're still the same person you were before you were a mum. Your world hasn't stopped because you've had a baby – you've just invited another person to share it with you.

2/ I WILL NOT PUNISH MYSELF FOR FINDING THINGS HARDER THAN BEFORE

After giving birth, when I couldn't even walk up the hill I used to sprint up, I broke down. I knew I was facing both a literal and metaphorical uphill struggle to get my body back to a fitness level I was comfortable with. I had to re-learn how my body worked while also looking after my mental health. That takes time and patience – which, for someone like me, was a huge learning curve. (Let's just say I'm not the most patient person in the world – I want everything yesterday, especially when waiting for food in the microwave!) We've become accustomed to instant satisfaction, with everything available at the click of a button or a swipe of our thumb, so not being able to order a 'feel top-notch again' miracle cure online sucks. But it took nine months to grow your baby: it'll take at least that long again to recuperate and find a new groove. Accept that, embrace it and enjoy the journey.

3/ I WILL LISTEN TO MY BODY

Write this commandment in a notebook or on your mirror in lipstick. You can even get it tattooed on your arm if necessary (I'm kidding, and I will not be held liable if you actually do, BTW). What I'm not kidding about is that this is one of the most important lessons in the whole book: you must listen to your body. Is it sore, tired, achy, hurting, bleeding, full, hungry, dehydrated, bloated or injured? If so, what does it want or need? Experiencing pregnancy and birth forces us to confront the reality of our physicality – a lesson we should continue to pay attention to postpartum. Starting a training plan means becoming aware of your body on a moment-by-moment basis, tuning into its likes and dislikes, learning when to up the

ante or when to lay off, and respecting, not ignoring, what it's telling you. You only get one body: look after it, and it'll look after you.

4/ I WILL ASK FOR HELP WHEN I NEED IT

I'm fiercely independent and have always found it hard to ask for help. Ever since I was a kid 'helping' my dad and grandad build the Caterham Super 7 sports cars my dad raced, I've been the one mucking in and hustling. Yet, having Mia forced me to accept that sometimes I'm not Superwoman – and that's OK. I've learned that being able to ask for help is a sign of strength, not weakness. Having my mum to stay after the birth when Gorka was away touring was a godsend. And she wanted to help. We often think we're a burden on others when actually people love to feel useful and show they care. Gorka says I'm getting better at knowing my limitations (just don't ask him about that time I lifted loads of stuff into the attic alone rather than waiting for him...), but showing vulnerability is new to me and it's something I've had to learn. But if I can learn, so can you!

5/ I WILL NOT GIVE IN TO 'MUM GUILT'

One of the biggest emotional changes you'll experience upon giving birth is one of the least talked about: guilt. You'll feel guilty about everything: going to work, not going to work, having a night off, doing something for yourself, giving them a dummy, not giving them a dummy, forgetting their hat, dropping them off at your parents', wishing they'd go to sleep, enjoying yourself without them, not enjoying yourself without them and so on. Once you've stepped onto the guilt rollercoaster, it spins so fast it's impossible to get off, so the best thing you can do is acknowledge the feeling and ask yourself the following questions: 'What would I tell a friend who felt this way?' (because we're much kinder to others than we are to ourselves); 'Am I being fair to myself?' (answer – no); 'Would a man feel bad about this?' (answer – no again!). Then give yourself a goddamn break.

6/ I WILL NOT COMPARE MY BODY TO ANYONE ELSE'S

Comparison is the thief of joy. Comparing your body to anyone else's is incredibly damaging at any time, but it's especially dangerous after having a baby, when your body is a stranger to you. Standing next to Janette Manrara, a dancer on *Strictly*, I'd look like a drag queen. She is tiny – five foot one – and I'd look huge next to her. Same goes for Lucy Mecklenburgh. She had her baby after me and looks incredible, but I know we're built entirely differently. I can't and won't ever look like her, any more than she can or will ever look like me – and that's fine, because I love the way I look! Doing this programme has given me such a confidence boost that I'll happily refer to myself as a MILF any day! Please only compare Today-You with Yesterday-You. Do you feel healthier and stronger today than yesterday? If not, what can you do today to make Tomorrow-You feel better?

7/ I WILL NOT COMPARE MY MOTHERING SKILLS TO ANYONE ELSE'S

Everyone's got an opinion, just like everyone's got an arsehole – but you don't want to know about their arseholes, do you? In which case, why should you care about their opinion? Trust your own judgement as a mother and as a person. You can't please everyone, and nor should you want to. I could post the most innocuous picture of Mia on social media and get a barrage

of grief: 'She shouldn't be wearing/eating/saying/doing that, blah blah blah.' If I listened to every comment, I'd be paralysed with nerves about posting anything at all for fear of offending someone – and then I'd no doubt get: 'It's selfish of you not to post anything when we follow you.' Sigh. All of which means: IGNORE THE KNOW-IT-ALLS. Trust your instincts and only listen to people you respect. No one knows the full story, so have faith in yourself. You got this. My mum always tells me, 'If they don't know you personally, don't take it personally.'

8/ I WILL BE KIND TO MYSELF AND PRIORITISE MY WELLBEING

Wanting to look after yourself is not selfish. Wanting to feel good, healthy and strong is positive for both you and your family. It's good parenting to want to be able to play with your kids, to pick them up, swing them about and crawl after them without having a heart attack. It's also a solid life plan to aim to be around to play with your grandchildren. It's entirely admirable to want to feel confident appearing in photos or when walking around the poolside in a swimsuit. You're teaching your little one that body confidence and good mental health are aspirational attributes. So be kind to yourself, look after yourself and prioritise your own wellbeing. Make sure you're in the best possible physical and mental position to raise them right. It's easier to raise a strong child than repair a broken adult. So stop beating yourself up for everything, and instead high-five yourself for having got this far and for wanting to go further.

9/ I WILL SURROUND MYSELF WITH SUPPORTIVE PEOPLE

It's sad that I need to say this, but people may react negatively to you making positive changes in your life. Sometimes growth scares people. They might see your positive actions as a reflection of what they're not doing: 'If you're doing that and I'm not, what does that say about me?' (This can be especially true when it comes to not boozing, which is an essential part of this plan.) If you tell people that you're starting this plan and get comments like, 'Why do you want to change?' or 'You're boring now', please ignore them. Surround yourself with supportive, positive people while on this journey, distancing yourself from those that make you feel bad. Tell your loved ones what you're doing – you'll rely on their support – and support others in turn. The nay-sayers will soon pipe down once they see how great you feel (and if they don't, it may be time to reassess your relationship with them...). Soon it'll go from, 'Why are you doing that?' to 'How are you doing that?' Remember, true friends will support you – and, if they're anything like my friends, whenever you're off the booze, they'll rely on you as a taxi after a night out as well! (I'm cool with that, just as long as they puke out of the window rather than inside the car...)

10/ I WILL REMEMBER THE JOURNEY MY BODY'S BEEN ON

Your body is a miracle. Think of everything it's done for you already: it's got you to where you are today. It's half of your mum, half of your dad. It's picked you up when you've fallen down. It's got you from A to B, it's loved and lost, it's got you out of tricky situations and it's always tried its best. And, on top of all that, it's just created a human. What more does it have to do to get your respect?! We all need to up our gratitude game. It's time to pay our bodies back for everything they've been through by treating them well and looking after them. This means eating good food, training in a safe way and building up both physical and mental strength. This book is about investing in your own self-worth and learning to love and appreciate yourself so you can look forward to a bright, positive, exciting future. You and your body are hopefully going to be around together for a long time, so enjoy the ride!

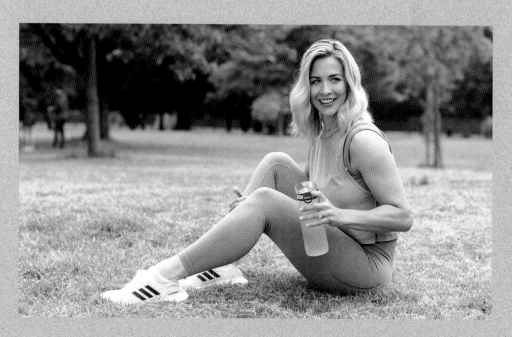

YOUR GOALS

Why did you pick up this book? What is it that you want to get out of this health and fitness journey? Where do you ideally see yourself in twelve weeks' time?

Before you start the plan, I'd like you to take a moment, alone, and copy out the Motivation Table opposite into a notebook and really consider your answers. Filling in this table might be the first time you've a) properly thought about exactly what you want to achieve, and b) spent time assessing your own motivations. It's a chance to be really honest with yourself about what's driving you.

Why does this matter? For so many reasons! By writing down why you're doing the plan, you'll learn more about yourself. If the truth is that you're being pushed into training by a partner, or you're motivated by a desire to look like a celebrity, write that down! Be honest. There are no 'wrong' answers. It'll actually probably feel like a relief to admit it. Treat this as your 'feel-good confessions' diary.

What I'm absolutely convinced will happen, though, is that your motivations will change as you progress. You'll go from 'I want to look good for Mike' to 'I want to keep feeling stronger for myself', and from 'I want to look like celebrity A' to 'I want to be the best version of me'. Why? Because, in looking after yourself, you'll build your self-esteem. You'll feel stronger, healthier, more capable and more confident. You'll start being kinder to yourself, respecting your body for what it can do, not punishing it for what it does or doesn't look like. Your self-worth will improve and you'll be less likely to compare yourself unfavourably to others and you'll want to continue feeling that way for *you*.

Chances are you won't stick to the plan if you're doing it solely for other people, or for reasons that don't inspire you. You'll end up resenting the effort and give up. There's a difference between a challenge and a chore. If you're doing this for someone else, or to reach an impossible ideal, it'll feel like a chore. By its very definition, a chore is a drag – something we avoid, put off or dread doing. On the other hand, we are eager to take on challenges, viewing them as something that will enrich us. You can move the goalposts along the way as you progress, constantly pushing yourself to achieve what you want to. A challenge is a way of bettering yourself (which is not true of a chore), and that means that seeing it through is hugely rewarding. Viewing this plan as a chore would mean that,

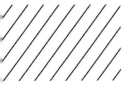

The yardstick of acceptability we measure ourselves against is always higher than that which we measure anyone else against.

Motivation Table

Date today	
When do you intend to start the plan?	
How do you feel about starting?	
Why are you starting this plan and what are your main goals? (*Be honest!*)	
How do you hope to feel physically at the end of the twelve weeks?	
How do you hope to feel mentally at the end of the twelve weeks?	
What are you most looking forward to experiencing on the journey?	
What are you least looking forward to going through/tackling on the journey?	
What stumbling blocks or obstacles do you think you might face?	
What solutions to these obstacles can you think of in advance?	
How will you reward yourself at the end of the twelve weeks?	
Rate how you feel about yourself now, on a scale of 1–10 (with 1 being 'I really don't like myself' and 10 being 'I'm basically Xena Warrior Princess').	

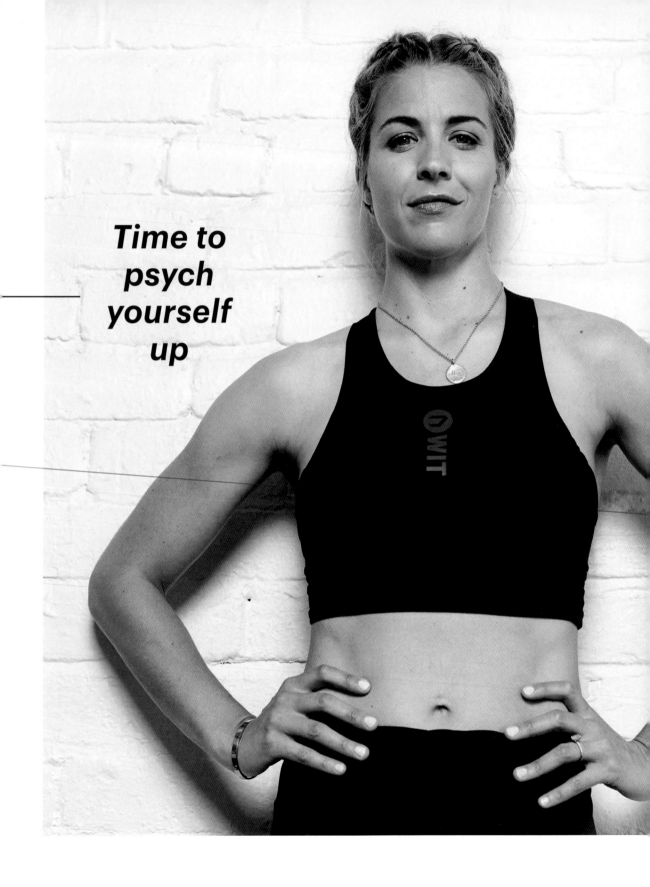

Time to psych yourself up

even if you did reach your goal (whatever it may be), you'd probably still feel unhappy. The yardstick of acceptability we measure ourselves against is always higher than that which we measure anyone else against. Filling out the Motivation Table will encourage you to consider more benefits and to think about the bigger picture: wouldn't it be fantastic to feel more energised? To learn how to cook quick, healthy meals? To discover new skills? To see what your body is capable of? To challenge yourself?

In the table, I also ask you to think about potential obstacles that may trip you up or that may offer you an excuse for quitting when things get tough! Identifying them now will give you more options for overcoming them and seeing them as challenges rather than deal-breakers. A 100-metre hurdles runner knows that the hurdle bars are going to be in their way before they start the race. Of course, you may come across totally unexpected snags, but the more prepared you are at the start, the less likely it is that they'll knock you off your game.

Filling in the Motivation Table may reveal some uncomfortable truths, but that's the point. It'll make it all the sweeter when you come to fill in the Reflection Table at the end of the journey (see page 295) and compare the two to see how far you've come. It'll also be really interesting to see whether the things you thought you'd least enjoy were as bad as you'd imagined!

Also, writing things down by hand will not only force you to really consider your answers (there's no easy 'edit' or 'delete' options with a pen) but also help prove to yourself that you're taking this seriously. Many of us hand-write shopping lists or to-do lists because we know that way we're less likely to forget things – and more likely to get them done!

It's so important to take time to reflect at both the start the and end of any journey, so you can properly appreciate what you've achieved and learned. That's why there's a box asking what reward you'll give yourself when you complete the plan. This is an added incentive. An extra kick up the arse, if you will. Something to work towards and to look forward to. It could be a holiday/a new outfit/a bottomless brunch – or all of the above (how about wearing a new outfit to a bottomless brunch while on holiday? Just throwing it out there). It's up to you. Just make sure it's something totally awesome that you actually really want – because you'll have damn well earned it.

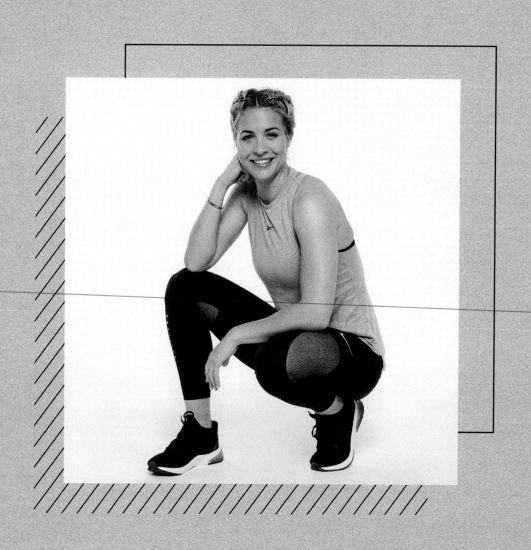

THE BABY STEPS BODY PLAN

WELCOME TO THE BABY STEPS BODY PLAN

Welcome to your new twelve-week training plan, created in partnership with my good friend and training buddy Olly Foster. Olly and I have known each other, personally and professionally, for more than eight years. He is a hugely successful personal trainer with over twenty years' experience in the industry, and he helps clients (both in person and online) to improve the way they feel, move and look. I trust him and his expertise implicitly. We created the first *Ultimate Body Plan* training programme together in 2018, and I'm thrilled to have him back on board for our new 'Baby Steps Body Plan'.

While the plan has been designed for women who want to get back to their best after having a baby, it will also help anyone looking for a gentle introduction – or reintroduction – to fitness. For the new mums, though, there are some essential things to bear in mind before starting this programme.

You are not in the same physical shape as you were before having a baby. No one expects you to be – you've just housed a tiny human for nine months! With that in mind, you need to be absolutely certain you're OK to start training. Typically speaking, new mums can start exercising six weeks after giving birth. However, if, like me, you had a caesarean, it can be more like twelve weeks. (I actually waited fifteen weeks, because I listened to my body and that's what felt right for me – see page 45.) During that time, breathing exercises and gentle walks are all that's recommended, unless you've been told differently by your aftercare team. Whether your baby 'came out of the sunroof or the boot', as one of my nurses put it, everyone's rate of recovery is entirely personal, so whatever your situation, it's essential you get the nod from your health worker or GP before you start.

You'll find the following information within this introduction:

- the nuts and bolts of the plan: what it is and how it works (pages 56–65)
- an explanation of why we're focusing on the core and pelvic floor (pages 66–69)
- tips on staying motivated and getting the most out of your workouts (pages 70–73)
- your Progress Table, and why tracking your mood is a key part of this plan (pages 74–75)

Trust the process, listen to your body and enjoy yourself!

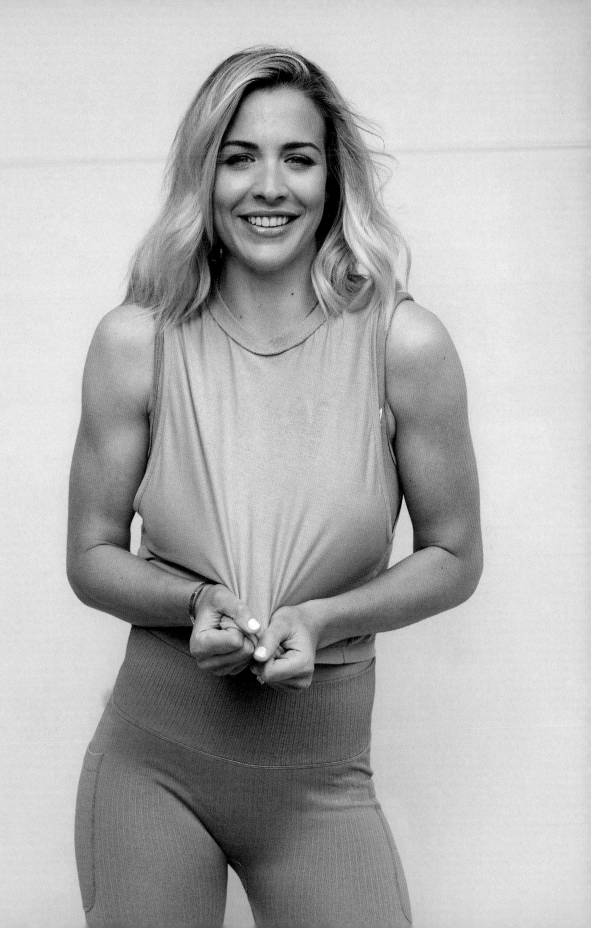

MEET YOUR NEW PLAN

The plan is split into three training phases of four weeks each (making twelve weeks altogether), and it gets progressively tougher as you do!

Ideally, you will complete four workout sessions a week: two strength sessions and two cardio/abs/core (CAC) sessions. For best results, you'll need to also stick to a healthy diet (see the food and recipe section on pages 132–275). Sadly, scarfing takeaways and drinking all the wine won't help you get the best from your workouts. Sorry.

Within each phase, you'll find four different workouts to choose from: two full-body strength workouts (one gym-based and one home-based) and two CAC workouts (one gym-based and one home-based). It's up to you whether you wish to train at home, in the gym or a combination of both. After the last couple of years we've all lived through, though, I highly recommend getting out of the house if you can! While training in the gym can seem intimidating to those not used to it, the camaraderie and friendships I've found working out among others can't be beaten. Remember, you can always ask a member of the gym staff to help you set up the equipment. They'll be happy to assist you. An example week on the plan will look like this:

Monday	Strength workout (gym or home)
Tuesday	CAC workout (gym or home)
Wednesday	Rest day
Thursday	Strength workout (gym or home)
Friday	CAC workout (gym or home)
Saturday	Rest day
Sunday	Rest day

Trying to squeeze in four workouts a week may sound like a lot, especially if having a shower and getting dressed feel like monumental achievements right now. But don't panic! If you manage two or three workouts a week while also staying consistent with your diet, you'll still make progress. It may take a bit longer, but it will still happen. While this is designed as a twelve-week plan, it's not a race. You can complete it in twenty, thirty or forty weeks. Listen to your body. If it's responding well after four weeks, move on to the next phase. If it's not, stick to what you're doing for a while until you feel ready to move on. And there doesn't need to be an end date to this. Once working out becomes part of your routine, you'll look forward to it (trust me!), and training will just become something you do, to the point where it would feel weird not making time to do it.

WHY & HOW THE PLAN WORKS

Short and sweaty

We know you're busy (understatement of the year), so each session should only last around thirty minutes:

<u>Warm-up</u>: 5 minutes / <u>Workout</u>: 20 minutes / <u>Cool-down</u>: 5 minutes

However, when you're just starting out and getting into the flow of things, the sessions may take a bit longer, especially if the exercises are new to you or if you need longer rest periods between each one. As you get stronger and the movements become more familiar, you'll find you get through each session a little faster.

You may notice some sessions instruct you to do fewer exercises than others. This is no indication of difficulty – it's because some muscles need to work harder than others. You'll find you're just as sweaty after a four-exercise session as after a six-exercise session.

Follow the leader

Complete the workouts (and phases) in the order they're presented, rather than jumping about from one exercise to another. Every workout is designed according to 'stimulation and adaptation', meaning each muscle is warmed up so it works to its full advantage, rather than being worked 'cold'. Picking exercises to do randomly (or jumping from phase to phase) won't only mean not getting the full effect of the workout – it could cause injury.

TRAINING AFTER A CAESAREAN

Caesareans (often referred to as 'C-sections') are relatively common nowadays, but that doesn't mean they're not a big deal. Everyone's situation is different, and the type of surgery and how it's performed is dependent on varying factors, but it will generally involve two incisions (one on your lower abdomen, below the bikini line, and one on your uterus), leaving you with two wounds that need to heal, both internally and externally. It is essential you give yourself time to rest and recover. Making sure you heal properly at the start will save you time, pain and complications in the future. Always check with your health worker or GP before starting to exercise. They will probably recommend waiting for at least twelve weeks((and you'll also need to avoid driving and heavy lifting for six weeks, or until signed off by your GP). I waited fifteen weeks before exercising, and even then I was only walking about pushing the pram.

THE STRENGTH WORKOUTS

This plan includes strength-training workouts (i.e. workouts using weights).

Now, before you freak out at the prospect of using weights, please remember: YOU WILL NOT 'HULK UP' FROM LIFTING WEIGHTS! Women don't have enough testosterone to get huge. It's hard enough for guys, let alone ladies! When practised in conjunction with cardio, all that lifting weights will do is get you sculpted, lean and – best of all – STRONG.

For your two strength sessions a week, you can choose either the gym-based workout, or the home-based one, or mix and match both. In the gym, you'll be using a mixture of free weights and resistance machines. For the home-based strength sessions, though, I recommend investing in a set of resistance bands. They are effective, inexpensive and readily available online. Get a set that includes different levels of tension and both 'closed' circular bands and ones with 'ends' or handles. You can use dumbbells instead of bands if you have them – just amend the exercises as you go. You'll notice some of the strength exercises don't mention using any weights or resistance at all. That's because you'll be using your body weight as the 'load' instead. For example, when doing a plank, your arms, feet and core 'lift' the weight of your body. *You*, effectively, are the weight. Which leads us neatly on to...

Get a load of this

You may hear the word 'load' a lot in the gym: it refers to the amount of weight lifted during an exercise. I can't tell you what weight is right for you, as it depends on lots of different factors. But here's a good general rule to follow when working with weights: pick what you think is a good starting weight and then work to the rep (repetition) range set and see how you feel, giving yourself a five-rep leeway. So, if the target number of reps for an exercise is ten to fifteen, but you find you can't get to ten reps without failing, the load is too heavy. However, if you find you can get to more than fifteen reps without failing, the load is too light. It's wise to start light and add weight, rather than start heavy and risk injury (and disappointment). Remember: it's not a competition!

It's also important to remember that some days you'll be stronger than others. One day you might feel like Wonder Woman, throwing around heavy-duty dumbbells, while the next you can barely lift them. Accept this as a fact of life. Don't beat yourself up; just work as hard as you can based on how you feel at the time. The golden rule is: NEVER sacrifice form for weight! If you can't maintain your lifting form (technique) throughout the set, reduce the weight (or the tension of the resistance band) until you can.

CAC WORKOUTS

The CAC workouts consist of cardio, ab and core exercises (I will explain more about core work on page 67).

Again, you'll complete two of these sessions each week, choosing either gym-based or home-based workouts, or mixing and matching the two. As this plan is designed for new mums, all of the exercises will initially be low impact, limiting any strain on the body (it has just been through a lot, to be fair). These exercises will increase in difficulty as you progress through the plan – but I can't reiterate enough how important it is to listen to your body. Do not progress and do not push yourself if you're not ready.

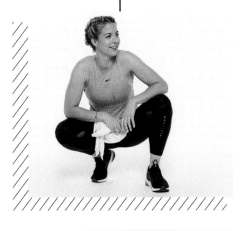

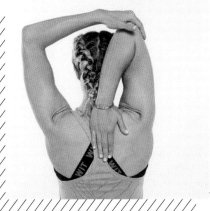

WARMING UP AND COOLING DOWN

Warming up and cooling down is imperative to this plan, and must be completed before and after EVERY workout. You've essentially been lugging a bowling ball about in your belly for nine months. It was then removed and handed to you to lift, cradle, cuddle and entertain. (That analogy got weird really quickly.) In short: your posture is probably shot to shit. You may be experiencing muscle tightness, hunched shoulders and a sore lower back. Sleepless nights and added stress don't help. Stretching, therefore, both before and after training, is your friend: it readies your body to work out, aids you in recovery and reduces your risk of injury.

For the warm-ups, we will be doing dynamic pre-exercise stretches. These literally warm up your muscles, deepening the stretch when muscles are tight to limit the risk of over-extending. The cool-down, meanwhile, makes the most of your limbered-up self to increase flexibility, decrease muscle aches and joint stress, and preserve muscle function. Aim to hold your cool-down stretches for fifteen to thirty seconds on each side, and don't forget to marvel at the fact that now you can not only see your toes, but also almost touch them.

FORM & TECHNIQUE

\ Good form versus bad form

'Good form!' sounds like something politicians shout during Prime Minister's Questions. It's actually personal-trainer speak for executing an exercise properly. Having 'good form' means following the instructions exactly, fully focusing on the task at hand and concentrating on the muscle you're working. 'Bad form' (wonky arms, a crooked back, etc.) means you risk not only seriously injuring yourself, but also wasting your time with a half-arsed workout.

Good form is especially relevant to new mums. Throughout pregnancy, women compensate for the physical changes they experience by moving in different ways. (I really missed sleeping on my tummy!) Muscles are tightened and stretched, and your body can fall out of alignment. Make sure you practise good form throughout the plan. If you feel unable to do so, are severely out of alignment, or find that you are leaking urine or experiencing pain or bleeding, please speak to your health worker or GP.

\ Tempo

'Tempo' is another key term and concept to keep in mind when training. It refers to the speed at which a movement is completed. Most beginners are so focused on performing the exercise correctly that they don't even think about the speed they're doing it at. Using the correct tempo improves body awareness and joint stability in and around the working muscle. It also strengthens connective tissue, and strengthens and engages the muscle more effectively. For every exercise in this plan, I would like you to use a controlled tempo all the way through the movement, pausing at both the top and the bottom of each rep. No speeding up when you're near the end of your rep count!

\ Use full ROM (range of motion)

I want you to punch the air with one fist right now. Go on, do it; I'll wait. Now look at your arm: it should be perfectly straight, with no bend at the elbow. If that describes your arm, congrats: you have completed the exercise using 'full ROM'. This means extending your limbs and muscles as fully as possible throughout the movement, with nothing impeding or restricting you. Fully extending, stretching and pushing leads to better results. During your workouts, therefore, please read the instructions and always try to use full ROM.

However, don't overdo it if you have a current or old injury – if you need to, you can reduce the range to suit you personally. For example, with a reverse lunge, if you're struggling to get your back knee close to the floor during the movement, only go down as far as you comfortably can.

\ Reps, sets and rest

The number of 'reps' (repetitions) called for is how many times you should complete an exercise, while a 'set' is a group of reps. For example, you may be instructed to 'complete three sets of fifteen reps'. In this plan, you'll be given either a target number of reps to hit (e.g. '10–15 reps on each arm') and a number of sets, or a target time period (e.g. 'complete alternate toe touches for 30 seconds'). You will also be allocated set rest periods. Based on your current level of fitness and how much time you have, you can increase or decrease rest periods, sets or reps. However, make sure you still do all of the exercises in order, so the muscles are suitably warmed up. And please be realistic about potential progress if you consistently minimise the amount you do.

Supersets
A superset is two different exercises performed concurrently without a rest between them. They're a great way to get the most out of your workout in a shorter amount of time. You'll find them throughout the plan, where they are marked as 'S/S'. If you do wish to superset your workout, wherever S/S is marked, you can move straight from that exercise to the next one.

\ Breathing

When diligently counting reps or trying to manoeuvre your legs behind your head (don't worry, that's not in the plan… or is it?!), it's common to hold your breath, or even forget to breathe altogether. But breathing properly is one of the most important aspects of form and technique (and also of, you know, staying alive). Knowing when to inhale and exhale not only deepens your stretches and improves your blood circulation, but is also very mindful. Focusing on your breathing anchors you in the present, calms down your busy head and makes you more aware of what you're doing.

When performing a strength-based exercise, unless stated otherwise, you should generally inhale during the relaxation phase and exhale during the exertion phase. Using a squat as an example, that means breathing in through your nose on the way down, then breathing out through your mouth on the way up.

MUSCLE GROUPS

If you've ever heard people talking about lats and glutes and obliques and wondered what they were on about, wonder no more. Because I'll be referring to different muscle groups in the workout section, here's a brief breakdown of what (and where) they all are so you can understand exactly which muscles the different exercises are working.

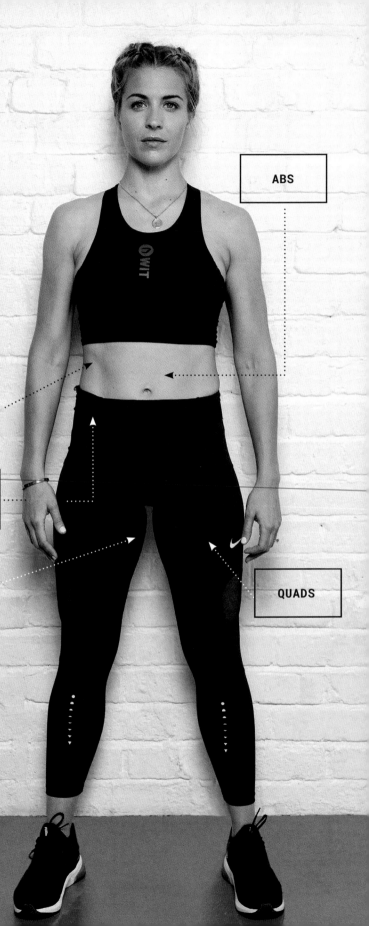

ABS

OBLIQUES

HIP FLEXORS

ADDUCTORS

QUADS

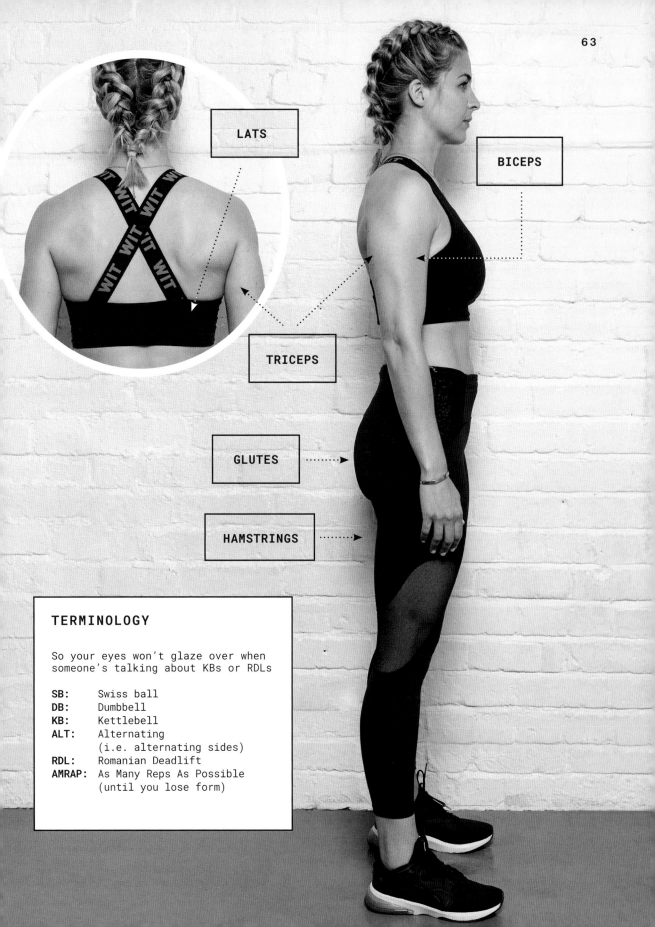

LATS

BICEPS

TRICEPS

GLUTES

HAMSTRINGS

TERMINOLOGY

So your eyes won't glaze over when someone's talking about KBs or RDLs

SB: Swiss ball
DB: Dumbbell
KB: Kettlebell
ALT: Alternating
(i.e. alternating sides)
RDL: Romanian Deadlift
AMRAP: As Many Reps As Possible
(until you lose form)

MUSCLE SORENESS OR DOMS

(delayed onset muscle soreness)

DOMS is the name for the aching experienced after training: when you walk like you've shat yourself, scream while trying to take off a jumper and can't actually bear the thought of climbing any stairs.

Experiencing aches and pains after exercising following a period of no exercise is totally normal and expected. DOMS is the result of tiny tears in the muscle fibres that can occur when they're strained. It hurts, sure, but it's not dangerous – it's part of the natural process of making your muscles work harder. Training with DOMS is fine – the more you work out, the more your muscles will strengthen, and the less DOMS you'll experience. Walking, stretching and using a foam roller can help with the aching and speed up recovery.

Please don't judge the quality of your workout on how much you ache afterwards. Not aching doesn't mean you weren't working hard enough – it means you're getting stronger!

SOME OTHER THINGS TO BEAR IN MIND

Relaxin
When I say 'relaxin', I'm not talking about 'Netflix and chill'! I'm talking about the hormone relaxin, which is produced by the ovary and placenta and causes ligaments and joints to 'relax' in preparation for childbirth. It can take months for joints to return to their previous levels of stability, so please take this into consideration when training, as you'll be more prone to injury. Be careful and watch your form.

Exercising while breastfeeding
Exercising does not impact your milk supply, so it's absolutely fine to take part in this programme while breastfeeding. However, do make sure you stay extra hydrated and be aware of the additional calories you'll require (we'll discuss both of these things in the recipe section – see page 136).

REST DAYS

Sorry, reader, but you're not a soldier (unless you actually are — in which case, bravo!). But even then, you still need rest days.

The strongest, fittest, most kickass women on the planet need rest days. Even Jet from Gladiators ('You will go on my first whistle' — who's with me?!) needs rest days. When training, your body goes through a lot: muscle tissue breaks down, muscle glycogen stores are depleted, there's fluid loss (through sweat), and your nervous, cardiovascular and musculoskeletal systems are all challenged. Your body, quite frankly, is FREAKING OUT.

Rest days give your body a chance to repair and recuperate. Energy stores and fluid levels are replenished, muscle tissue is repaired, the nervous system regenerates and your mind is given time and space to reflect. Rest days allow you to adapt and become stronger. Do not kid yourself that pushing too hard is beneficial — it will backfire. Please stick to having three days off a week. Well, you're a parent, so you never get a 'day off', but you know what I mean!

THINGS YOU CAN DO ON YOUR REST DAYS

- A gentle walk with your baby in the pram.

- Some foam rolling exercises if you're sore.

- Practise the warm-up and cool-down components of the plan — but no workouts!

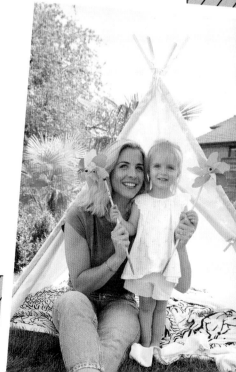

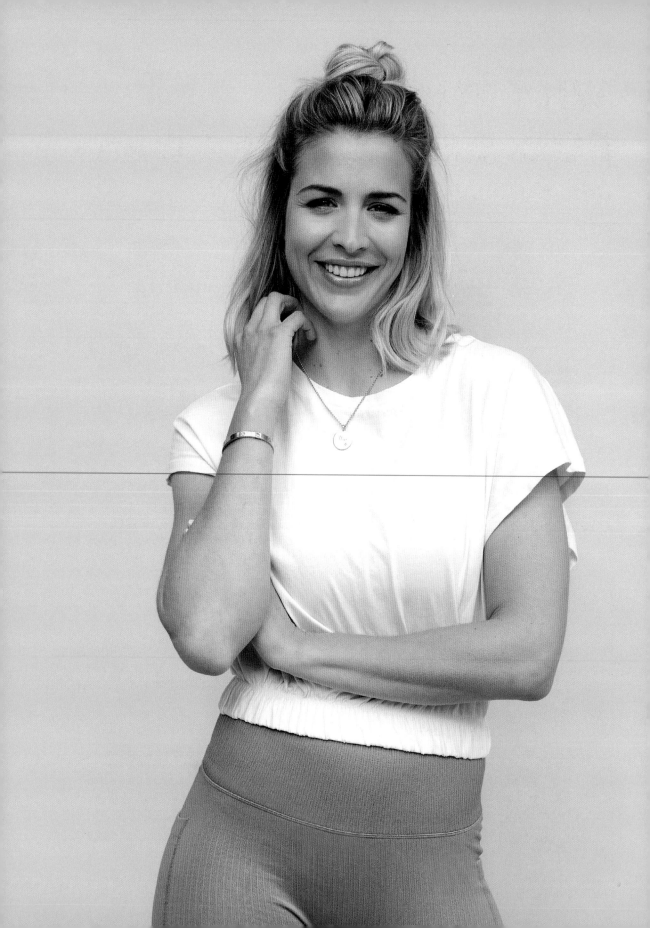

WHY THE PLAN FOCUSES ON THE CORE
(and the pelvic floor!)

'The core' is the umbrella term for a group of muscles: your pelvic floor, abdominals, back muscles and diaphragm (breathing muscle).

Imagine your body is a watch (bear with me here) and you open the back. The core would be a big cog made up of lots of smaller cogs. If one of the smaller cogs gets damaged, it affects how the whole machine works. The core is just that: the core of the body's muscular function. It's responsible for how well you perform everyday tasks. Unfortunately, your abdominals and pelvic floor are put under a great deal of strain and stress during pregnancy and birth. This training plan, therefore, has a strong focus on building up core strength as a whole, and pelvic floor strength in particular.

Why you may get a 'mummy tummy' or 'pooch'

As your pregnancy progresses, your abdominals stretch and your back muscles shorten. Once you've given birth, most women will experience some form of abdominal separation (mine was 4cm). Most of these gaps close of their own accord within four to twelve weeks. However, when the gap is roughly 2.7cm or larger, it's called diastasis recti – which is as un-fun as it sounds.

What is diastasis recti?
Diastasis recti (DR) is the separation of your 'six-pack' muscles. The natural gap between the two long parallel muscles on the left and right of your torso widens down the middle during pregnancy, causing your stomach to stick out between the gap, forming what's commonly known as a 'mummy tummy' or 'pooch'. The main symptom is a bulge in your stomach, especially when you strain or contract your abs. Additional symptoms include:

- **Lower-back pain:** When the abdominal wall is weak and DR creates more disconnection, the spine can feel unsupported, leading you to hunch or stand with bad posture. This contributes to an achy lower back.
- **Bloating:** If you have DR, bloating feels more obvious, as you have less support from the weakened abdominal wall and connective tissue. This can lead to your 'pooch' becoming more pronounced.
- **Pelvic floor issues:** See page 68.

How do I know if I have DR? And is it safe to exercise if I do?

If you suspect you have DR, please speak to your health worker about how to check and what that means for you personally. Depending on how wide your separation is, you may be referred to a physical therapist for a rehab plan, and you must then seek approval from the therapist before starting this programme. Unfortunately, most of the exercises here consist of movements that may make your DR worse if you start too soon.

Your (poor) pelvic floor

Your pelvic floor is stretched during pregnancy due to the weight of your baby, and the pelvic floor muscles also relax with hormonal changes in pregnancy. They are then put under even more strain during a vaginal birth (especially during an assisted vaginal birth, e.g. with forceps). Symptoms of a weak pelvic floor include urinary incontinence (leaking wee during the day, especially when laughing, coughing or exercising), breaking wind and even soiling yourself.

This is because it's harder to squeeze the muscles and sphincters at the bottom of the bladder or anus. You may also experience a 'heavy' sensation around your bottom half. This is because your bladder, bowels and uterus aren't being properly supported.

If any of these symptoms sound familiar, please see a personal trainer or physiotherapist who specialises in pelvic floor and core rehabilitation. The exercises within our training plan will help, but you may also need more personalised treatment. It's important that pelvic floor exercises are done regularly – you could try to get into the habit of doing them at a particular time every day, for example when you're folding laundry or browsing Instagram.

What exactly is your pelvic floor?

Your pelvic floor is a web of muscles, ligaments and tissues stretched across your pelvic bones. It supports your:

* womb (uterus)
* vagina
* bladder
* bowels

Think of it like a trampoline, stretching and bouncing in response to added pressure, weight or movement.

Its job is to:
* support pelvic organs and other abdominal contents
  (i.e. digestive organs)
* support the growing baby in pregnancy
* help maintain continence
* help prevent prolapse

HOW TO ENGAGE YOUR CORE

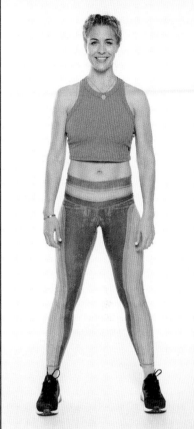

I want you to engage your core before EVERY exercise you do on this plan. Engaging your core not only increases core strength, but also helps to maintain form and so reduces the risk of injury.

HERE'S HOW TO DO IT:

1/ Inhale deeply through your nose so you can feel your ribcage, stomach and pelvic floor gently expand.

2/ Breathe out through your mouth. As you exhale, forcefully contract your abs as if you are bracing for a punch to the stomach. You should be aiming to create that tight feeling of trying to stop yourself from peeing, or the sensation you get when you cough or laugh (it can help to purse your lips). Doing this will activate the pelvic floor and transverse abdominal muscle (TVA), the deepest layer of your abdominal muscles.

3/ Another way to do it is to rest your hands on the sides of your stomach and attempt to push them away using only your abs.

Once you have engaged your core, you should still be able to breath naturally. Continue to engage for the duration of the exercise. It will take practice to get it right, and to get used to it, so please try to engage your core whenever you remember at random times during the day — and always engage before picking up your baby.

TRACKING YOUR PROGRESS

If you follow this plan while maintaining a balanced diet, your body will change. It will get stronger, leaner and more sculpted. You will be able to lift more, you'll enjoy more flexibility and you'll have more stamina (which you'll need for all that 3 a.m. please-go-to-sleep-for-the-love-of-God rocking). Wanting to see those changes is entirely valid and motivational.

But please don't turn to the scales to track how you're doing – weight loss is not a good indication of progress, and monitoring it can be detrimental to your mental health. Women can lose around 13lbs (5.6kg) during childbirth. That includes the baby (obvs), the placenta and amniotic fluid. During the first week after birth, you'll also lose retained fluids. However, any fat gained or stored won't just disappear. Lots of other things can affect your weight, especially after pregnancy, including water retention, periods and hormonal changes. In addition, building your muscles can actually mean putting on weight. Stepping on the scales can be an emotional minefield, determining how you feel all day. This isn't healthy or productive. Therefore, on my plan, scales are banned. Instead, if you'd like to monitor your progress, please use these alternative methods.

Weekly photographs

Every Monday morning, take a photo of yourself in your underwear. Take it at the same time and place every week. Make sure there's good lighting and that you take the photo before you eat or drink anything. Don't be self-conscious – these photos are for you and you alone. You may not like what you see, but you should! Your body has done miraculous things and you should love every bump, lump and stretch mark. What's more, your body is going to change – and seeing that progression will be really cool. We don't tend to notice changes in ourselves (or in other people who we see every day), so these photos will be a big pat on the back for future-you.

Measure yourself and pay attention to how your clothes fit

Measure your hips, waist, mid-thighs and upper arms with a tape measure once a week and write down the results. (It makes sense to do this after taking the photo, so it all becomes part of your routine.) You'll lose inches from some places, and it's motivational to see those figures in black and white. Also, pay attention to how your clothes are fitting – trousers, dresses and skirts becoming roomier are a sure sign things are changing.

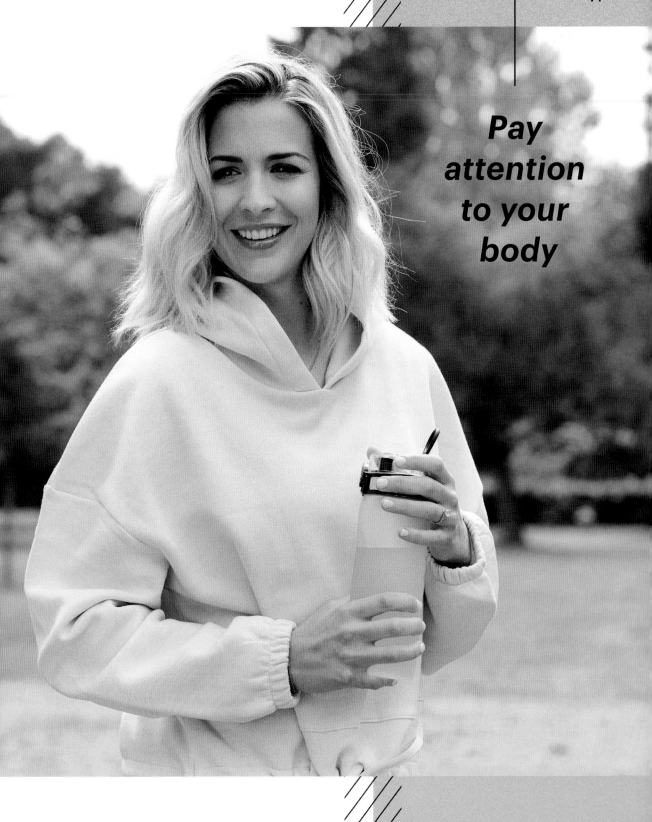

Pay attention to your body

THINGS TO BEAR IN MIND WHEN TRAINING

1/ SLEEP – WHENEVER AND HOWEVER YOU CAN

Chance would be a fine thing, huh? I know, I know – sleep is probably a touchy subject right now, but it's so important for both mental and physical health – especially when training – that it would be remiss of me not to mention it here. Sleep is when your body replenishes energy and repairs muscles, cells and tissues. If you don't get enough, your workouts will suffer, as will your post-training recovery time. In fact, sleep is such a big deal, I've dedicated a whole section to it in the wellbeing chapter – see pages 286–287.

2. EXERCISING SHOULD MAKE YOU FEEL ENERGISED, NOT DEPLETED

There's a difference between tiredness and fatigue. Upon finishing a workout, feeling tired is totally normal. Feeling completely emotionally and physically drained, however, is not. Feeling tired is an appropriate physical response after an active day. You can feel tired but still be proud of yourself and buzzing that you had a good workout. When I say fatigue, I mean a full-body exhaustion that a good night's sleep won't cure.

Look after yourself: if training isn't making you feel good, energised and positive but run-down, exhausted and knackered, speak to your health worker or GP about whether it's too early to start training, and if there might be anything underlying going on.

3. DON'T COMPARE YOUR TRAINING REGIME TO OTHERS'

Comparison (and what a bastard it is) is something I also talk about on page 46. However, it's important to say it here, too. When it comes to training, please don't compare your progress to anyone else's. Everyone is different – especially now. Some people will have had straightforward births, some people will have had awful births (*raises hand*). Some people will have trained hard before getting pregnant, so muscle memory will help them out. Some people's hormones will balance back out super fast, while others' will continue to go haywire for months. All of which means that comparing your workout regime to anyone else's is unproductive, as is comparing your physical progress with theirs. Don't do it to yourself. If you find social media a dispiriting place to be, you're looking at the wrong accounts and you're telling yourself the wrong narrative.

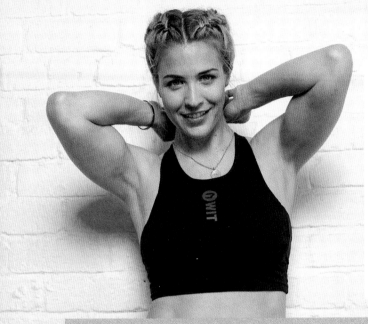

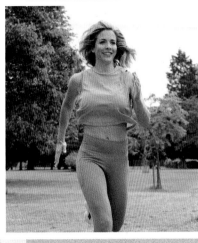

4. BE KIND TO YOUR BODY

There is no quick fix. No magic potion that will take your body back to what it once was. It took nine months to grow your baby (or ten, depending on who you speak to), so to expect it to just magically 'snap back' to the way it was before is damaging and unrealistic. Don't forget: your body GREW ANOTHER HUMAN BEING AND THEN EITHER BIRTHED IT OR HAD SURGERY. GIVE IT A BREAK.

I sometimes think that because having a baby is so natural, and because so many people do it, we forget that it's still a physical trauma. Not only that, but also your hormones are all over the shop and sleep is non-existent. So, please listen to your body, respect it, and don't push it too hard too fast.

5. YOU ARE DOING MORE THAN YOU THINK

Cut yourself some slack. Being a new mum is overwhelming. The last thing you need to do is beat yourself up about missing a session or agonising over whether you could have done more. You're no doubt already familiar with mum guilt (see pages 45–46), so why pile more pressure on yourself? Just do what you can. The very fact you're even attempting the plan is bloody impressive. Also remember that just increasing your movement throughout the day is valuable. Non-exercise activity thermogenesis (NEAT) is the energy you expend doing stuff that's not strictly exercise, like housework, walking up and down the stairs, food shopping and so on. It all adds up. So, even if you do miss a workout, don't berate yourself. Instead, try to be super focused on the physical aspects of those other activities – for example, try to engage your core while walking, or lunge about while cooking. This will still have a big impact on improving your fitness.

YOUR PROGRESS TABLE

Monitoring your mood is a massively important part of this plan.

How you feel emotionally will affect everything: how motivated you feel to work out and eat well; how much effort you put into training, forward-planning and being kind to yourself; even how honest you are with yourself over the choices you make. If you feel low, anxious, worried, annoyed and frustrated, you're less likely to follow through on the commitments you made to yourself on page 49 (and now's a good time to re-read the table you filled in on that page). If you're not feeling good emotionally, you'll also be less likely to train (because why bother?), less likely to eat well (because I don't have time to cook, FFS) and less likely to look after yourself (because I'm not a priority).

When you introduce something new into your life that demands time, patience and sacrifice – like this plan – it's easy to blame it for any stress and anxiety you feel. It's new and it's a pain, therefore you'd be better off without it, right?

Wrong!

On the following page is your Progress Table. Draw it out in your notebook, and fill it in when you first wake up in the morning, and again in the evening, before you go to bed. You'll be making a note of your mood, but also how your body feels, what workout you do and what you eat. This way, you'll be able to see any patterns in how your mood influences your behaviour, and vice versa. If you feel miserable to begin with, are you more likely to skip training or eat badly? If so, how does that leave you feeling? If you do train, does it lift your mood, even if your body aches? Do you find you enjoy your food more on the days you work out?

Be honest with yourself: are you fully invested in this plan? If not, why not? Is there something else going on at a deeper level? Is it physical or mental? Filling in this table will help you to get to know yourself better – which is something to be proud of. I've filled in some example entries for you, to show you how you can use the table to keep track of all these things.

DATE	7 August	8 August	9 August	10 August
HOW I FEEL mentally & physically (morning)	**Body:** slow, sluggish **Mind:** determined	**Body:** strong **Mind:** positive	**Body:** exhausted after a bad night's sleep **Mind:** I can't be arsed!	**Body:** sore back **Mind:** anxious but determined
WORKOUT	Home strength workout	Gym CAC workout	REST DAY	Home CAC workout
BREAKFAST	Blueberry & peanut protein porridge	Avocado & spinach smoothie bowl	Turkish eggs	Portobello mushrooms on toast
LUNCH	Sweetcorn & spinach pancakes	Butternut squash soup	Fish finger wraps	Chunky veg soup
DINNER	Super-quick tofu noodles	Cauliflower carbonara	Speedy rice & prawns	Chickpea & mushroom burger
DESSERT	None	None	Orange choc & nut pots	Easy raspberry sorbet
SNACK/ DRINK	Fruit skewers	Green power smoothie	Chocolate, coconut & mango thins	None
HOW I FEEL mentally & physically (evening)	**Body:** achy **Mind:** happy, proud	**Body:** tired, in a good way **Mind:** worried about doctor's appointment tomorrow	**Body:** Full, uncomfortable **Mind:** Low	**Body:** strong **Mind:** felt so much better eating because I was hungry rather than stressed

YOUR WARM-UP

The warm-up and cool-down should take five minutes each — possibly a bit longer when you're first starting out — and should be completed before and after every single workout in each phase. As with all exercises in this plan, your core should be engaged throughout (see page 69).

EXERCISE	SETS	REPS/TIME	TARGET AREA
Hip-flexor dynamic stretch	1	10 reps per side	Hips/groin
Cat to dog (yoga buffs will know this as cat to cow)	1	10 reps total	Pelvis
Banded monster walks	1	5 reps each way x 2	Glute activation
Hamstring swing	1	10 reps per side	Hamstrings
Glute bridge into clam shells	1	10 reps of each	Glute activation
Pole squat hold	1	5 reps total	Hips and ankles

HIP-FLEXOR DYNAMIC STRETCH

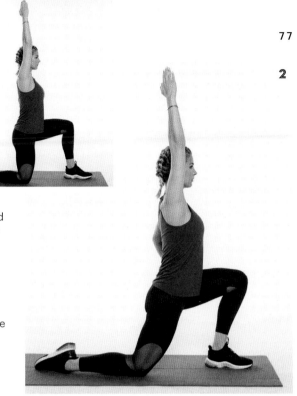

1 Kneel down on your right knee like you're about to propose to some lucky bugger. Your left foot should be planted firmly on the floor with the knee bent at a 90-degree angle. Extend your right arm straight up towards the sky.

2 With a neutral pelvis and straight back, push your left knee forwards over the toe line. Lean as far as you comfortably can until you feel a good deep stretch in your groin area. Hold for 2 seconds before returning to the starting position. Repeat 9 times, then swap sides.

CAT TO DOG

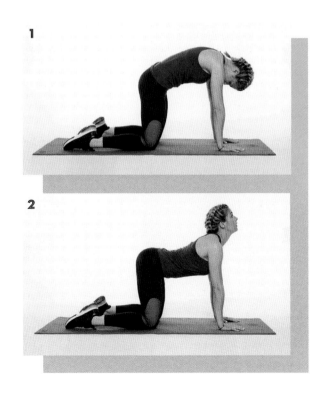

1 Get on your hands and knees, arms directly below shoulder joints and upper thighs below hip joints. Make sure there is an equal amount of weight placed across all points of contact with the floor. In a smooth movement, arch your back up towards the ceiling, sucking in your stomach and tucking your chin into your chest.

2 Once you have flexed as far as possible, arch the other way, so your stomach drops towards the ground. Lift your head up and squeeze your shoulders. Repeat this movement for the desired number of reps.

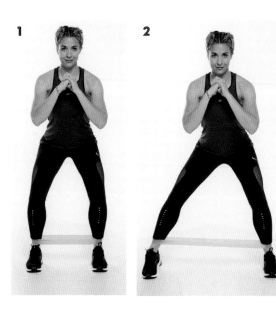

BANDED MONSTER WALKS

1 Loop a closed resistance band around your ankles and stand in an athletic position, as pictured.

2 Take a very small side step towards the right, stretching the band between your feet. Bring your left foot across to the right so your feet are back to hip-width apart. The band should stay taut the whole time. Repeat for a further 4 side steps before heading back to the starting position.

3 Once there, do the same as above but going forwards: a small step out and to the right, followed by a small step out and to the left. Repeat for 5 steps forward and 5 back, then repeat the whole circuit (side-to-side and forward-and-back) once more.

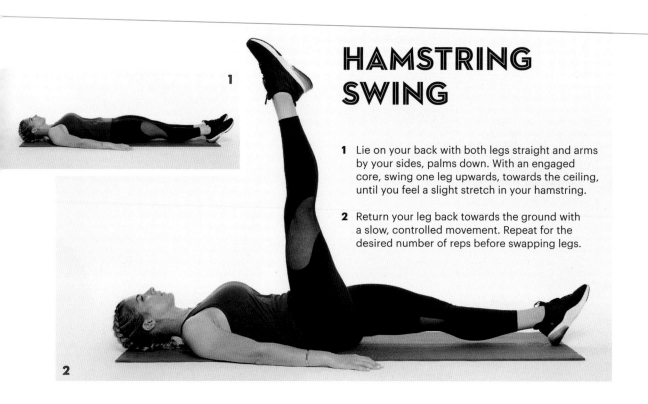

HAMSTRING SWING

1 Lie on your back with both legs straight and arms by your sides, palms down. With an engaged core, swing one leg upwards, towards the ceiling, until you feel a slight stretch in your hamstring.

2 Return your leg back towards the ground with a slow, controlled movement. Repeat for the desired number of reps before swapping legs.

The Baby Steps Body Plan

GLUTE BRIDGE INTO CLAM SHELLS

GLUTE BRIDGE

1 Lie on your back with a mini closed resistance band around your lower thighs (just above the knees). Your knees should be bent at a 45-degree angle, with your feet hip-width apart.

2 Lift your hips towards the ceiling, driving your weight through your heels, keeping tension on the band by pushing your knees out to the side and squeezing your glutes. Don't arch your lower back in this top position – just hold for a second while continuing to squeeze your glutes, making sure your body is in a straight line from knees to shoulders, and tucking your hips in.

3 Lower yourself back down to the starting position by rolling your spine slowly down from the top to bottom. Repeat 9 more times, then go straight on to clam shells.

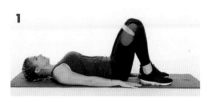

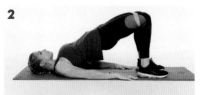

CLAM SHELLS

1 Keeping the band in exactly the same position, roll onto your right-hand side, with your hips, knees and ankles stacked on top of each other and your knees bent at a 90-degree angle.

2 Keeping your feet together, lift your left knee towards the ceiling (you should feel your outer glute working). Go as far as you comfortably can without leaning forwards or tipping backwards. Hold for a second, then slowly return to the starting position. Repeat 4 more times, then swap sides (so you'll complete 10 reps altogether).

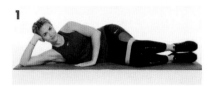

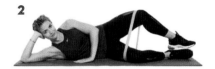

POLE SQUAT HOLD

1 This is a standard squat, but it uses a pole to assist you in getting into a full sitting position. (A staircase banister will also work.) Stand in front of the pole with your feet slightly wider than hip-width apart and your toes turned out. Clasp your hands around the pole.

2 Still holding the pole, drop into a squat position, keeping your torso straight. Try to sit deep into the squat without your heels lifting off the floor. Pause for 5 seconds at the bottom before slowly coming back up, then repeat 4 more times.

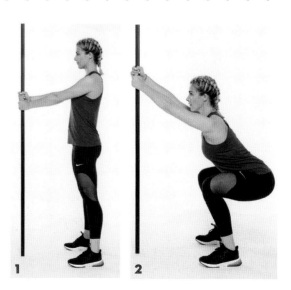

YOUR
COOL-DOWN

EXERCISE	SETS	REPS/TIME	TARGET AREA
Triceps stretch	1	15–30 seconds per arm	Triceps
Chest stretch	1	15–30 seconds	Shoulders
Quad stretch	1	15–30 seconds per leg	Quads
Hip-flexor stretch	1	15–30 seconds per side	Groin
Glute stretch	1	15–30 seconds per leg	Glutes
Hamstring stretch	1	15–30 seconds per leg	Hamstring

TRICEPS STRETCH

1 Stand upright, with your feet hip-width apart. Lift one arm above your head and bend the elbow to reach your hand down behind your neck towards your upper back – as if you need a good scratch.

2 Use your free hand to gently push down on the elbow to increase the stretch. Hold, then repeat on the opposite arm to complete 1 set.

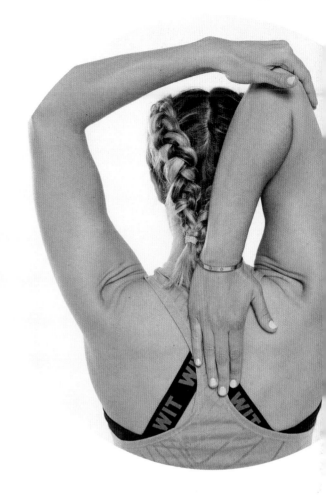

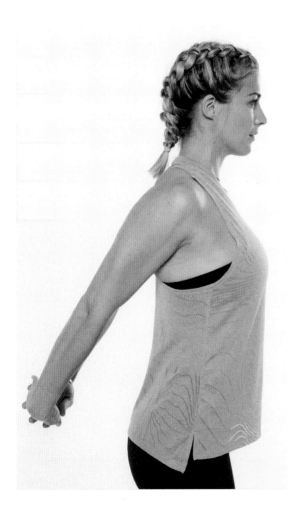

CHEST STRETCH

1 Stand upright, with your feet hip-width apart and your shoulders square but relaxed. Interlock your fingers behind your back, near your glutes.

2 Lift your arms slowly upwards, squeezing your shoulder blades together and keeping your back straight. Hold at your highest point, then return and release.

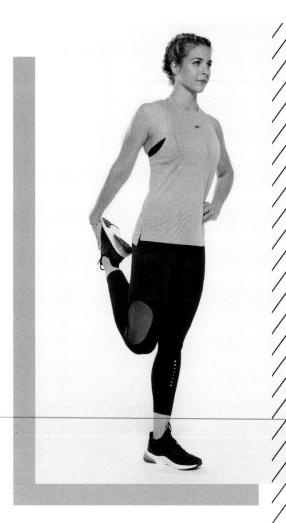

HIP-FLEXOR STRETCH

1 This is similar to the stretch in the warm-up – just without your arm in the air. Kneel down on your right knee with your left foot planted in front of you and the knee bent at a 90-degree angle. Keep your back straight.

2 From here, lean forwards through the hips to feel a stretch in the front of your right leg. Hold and repeat on the other side.

1

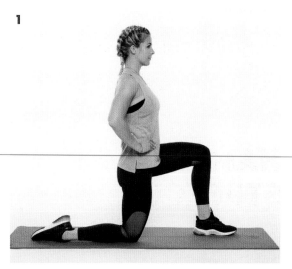

2

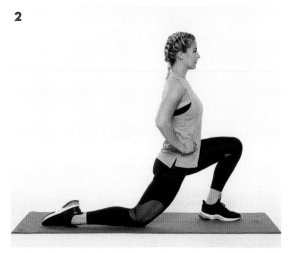

QUAD STRETCH

This is super simple: stand up straight and bend one of your legs up behind you, catching your ankle or foot with your hands and pulling it in towards your bum to increase the stretch. Make sure your pelvis is in a neutral position, and don't arch your back. You may need to hold on to a wall for balance. Hold and repeat with the other leg to complete 1 set.

GLUTE STRETCH

1

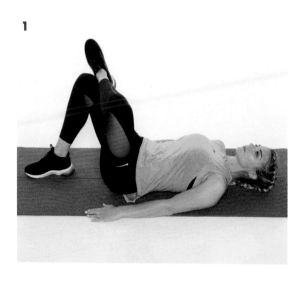

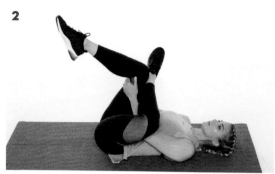

1 Lie on your back with your knees bent at a 45-degree angle and your feet flat on the floor. Lift your left foot up and rest it across your right knee.

2 Clasp your hands underneath the right thigh and pull it up towards your chest. You should feel a stretch in the outer glute of your bent leg. Hold and repeat on the other side for 1 set.

2

HAMSTRING STRETCH

1

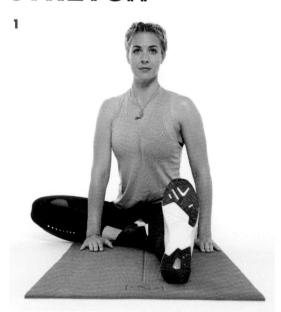

1 Sit on the floor with your left leg out straight in front of you and your right leg bent, with your right foot resting against the inside thigh of your left leg.

2 Lean your torso forwards over your left leg, holding on to that foot, if possible, to increase the stretch in your hamstrings. Hold, then repeat on the other side to complete 1 set.

2

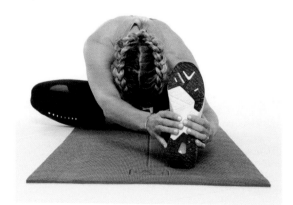

PHASE 1:
HOME STRENGTH WORKOUT

Warm-up (see page 76): **5 minutes**

Workout: **20–25 minutes**

Cool-down (see page 80): **5 minutes**

EXERCISE	SETS	REPS/TIME	REST	TARGET AREA
Hip thrusts	3	10–15 reps	(S/S)	Glutes and hamstrings
Resistance band kneeling shoulder press	3	10–15 reps per side	45 seconds	Shoulders and triceps
Resistance band squat to chair	3	10–15 reps	(S/S)	Full lower body
Resistance band face pulls	3	10–15 reps	45 seconds	Upper back and biceps
Prisoner reverse lunges	3	10–15 reps per side	(S/S)	Lower body (glutes and hamstrings)
Half kneeling resistance band chest press	3	10–15 reps per arm	45 seconds	Chest and triceps

HIP THRUSTS

SETS	REPS	REST
3	10–15 reps	(S/S)

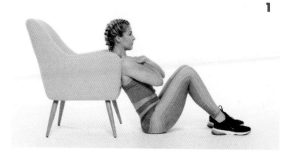

1 Sit on the ground with your shoulders leaning against the side of a sofa or chair, arms crossed over your chest. Bend your knees to a 45-degree angle, plant your feet firmly on the floor and engage your core.

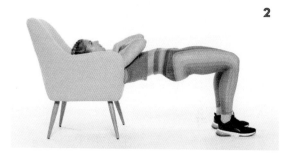

2 Inhale, then, on the exhale, drive your hips up towards the ceiling until your knees are bent at a 90-degree angle and your upper body forms a straight line, parallel to the floor. Pause at the top, squeeze your glutes, and slowly lower your bum back to the ground before repeating for the desired number of reps.

RESISTANCE BAND KNEELING SHOULDER PRESS

SETS	REPS	REST
3	10–15 reps	45 seconds

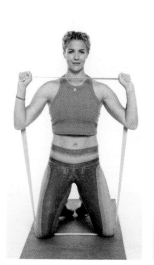
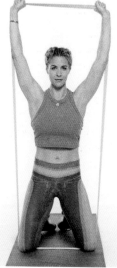

1 Kneel on one side of a closed resistance band with your knees hip-width apart. Then, with your palms facing towards the ceiling and shoulder-width apart, pull the other side of the band up to your shoulders (creating a square shape with the band).

2 Engage your core and drive your hands further up towards the ceiling, pulling the band taut. Maintain form: don't lean back or thrust your hips forwards. Pause at the top and return to the starting position, slowly and with control. Repeat for the desired number of reps. If this is too difficult, kneel on the band with only one knee and perform the same movement.

RESISTANCE BAND SQUAT TO CHAIR

SETS	REPS	REST
3	10–15 reps	(S/S)

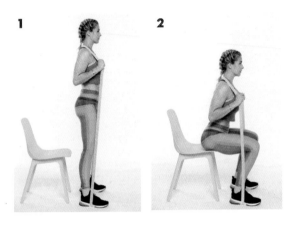

1 Stand on one side of the band with your feet shoulder-width apart and a chair behind you. Hook the other side of the band around your neck and grip it at shoulder height, with elbows tucked in.

2 Engage your core and bend your knees, sitting backwards towards the chair. Sit with your back straight and a slight forward lean. From there, stand back up by driving your weight through the middle of your feet. At the top, squeeze your glutes before repeating the movement.

* If the resistance is too easy, widen your feet a little to increase tension. If it's too hard, ditch the band and work with your body weight only.

RESISTANCE BAND FACE PULLS

SETS	REPS	REST
3	10–15 reps	45 seconds

1 Attach a resistance band (either closed or with ends) to a fixed anchor point at roughly shoulder height. Hold the other side (or ends) with an overhand grip, hands shoulder-width apart. Stand with one foot slightly in front of the other, with your back straight, arms fully extended and core engaged.

2 Pull your hands towards your ears as far as possible while keeping your palms facing down. Squeeze your upper back and shoulder blades together as you pull. Pause for a second, then return back to the starting position with a controlled movement. Repeat for the desired number of reps.

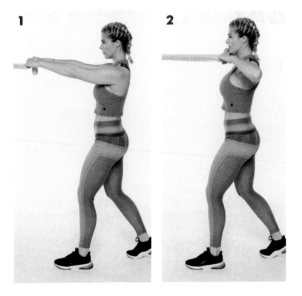

PRISONER REVERSE LUNGES

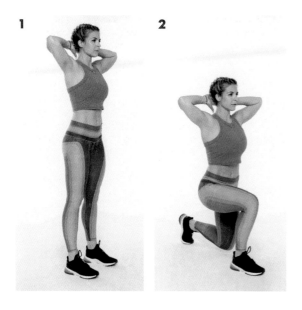

SETS	REPS	REST
3	10–15 reps per side	(S/S)

1 Stand with feet shoulder-width apart, hands clasped behind your neck, core engaged.

2 Step backwards with one leg, flexing the knee to drop the hips towards the ground. Continue the lunge until your rear knee nearly touches the floor, keeping your spine tall and the weight in your front foot towards the heel. Pause at the bottom before driving your weight back up through the heel of your front foot. Alternate legs for the desired number of reps.

* To increase difficulty, slow down the tempo and/or increase the number of reps.

HALF KNEELING RESISTANCE BAND CHEST PRESS

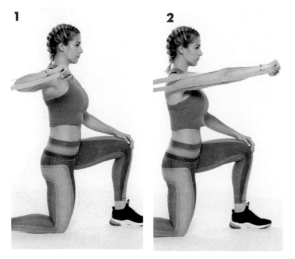

SETS	REPS	REST
3	10–15 reps per side	45 seconds

1 Attach a resistance band to a secure anchor point at roughly waist height. Facing away, hold the other end of the band in one hand and take a few steps forwards to increase the tension. Drop into a kneeling split stance (like you're going to propose), making sure the knee on the ground is the same side as the hand holding the band. Hold your arm as pictured.

2 Drive your arm forwards to extend the band out in front of you until your elbow nearly locks. Hold for a second, squeezing the chest and triceps, before slowly returning to the starting position. Repeat for the desired number of reps before swapping sides (both arm and leg) to complete one set.

PHASE 1:

HOME CAC (CARDIO, ABS & CORE) WORKOUT

Warm-up (see page 76): **5 minutes**

Workout: **20–25 minutes**

Cool-down (see page 80): **5 minutes**

EXERCISE	SETS	REPS/TIME	REST	TARGET AREA
Alternating toe touches	5	30 seconds	(S/S)	Glutes, hamstrings and core
Windmills	5	10 reps per side	45–60 seconds	Hips, legs and core
Kneeling Superman	4	5–10 reps per side	(S/S)	Glutes, lower back and core
Dead bugs	4	5–10 reps per side	30–45 seconds	Abs, core and posture
Resistance band anti-rotational step back	3	10 reps per side	(S/S)	Glutes, core and obliques
Hollow hold	3	5-second hold, 5 reps	30–45 seconds	Core and abs

ALTERNATING TOE TOUCHES

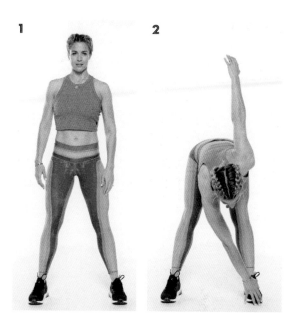

SETS	TIME	REST
5	30 seconds	(S/S)

1 Stand up tall with your chest proud, core engaged and arms down by your sides.

2 Bending from your hips and with your knees (don't lock them out), touch your left foot with your right hand. Rise up with a controlled movement, then repeat on the other side, touching your right foot with your left hand. Alternate sides for the set amount of time.

WINDMILLS

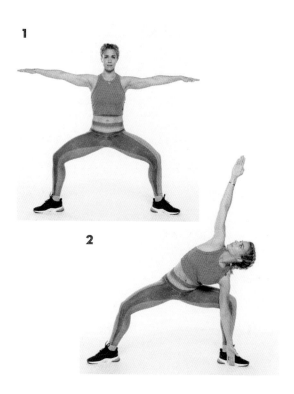

SETS	REPS	REST
5	10 reps per side	45–60 seconds

1 Set your feet wide in half squat position with your toes turned out. Extend your arms out on either side.

2 Reach one arm up towards the ceiling, with your upper body still facing forwards. Looking up at the hand that is reaching upwards, try to touch the floor with your other hand, without rounding the upper back. Only go as far as you comfortably can. Hold, then slowly return to the start position. Repeat nine times, then swap to the other side.

* If this is too easy, bring your feet closer together to shoulder width, keeping the legs straight, pushing the hips back, then repeat the same movement. You can also hold a water bottle in the extended arm to increase the load and make it more challenging.

KNEELING SUPERMAN

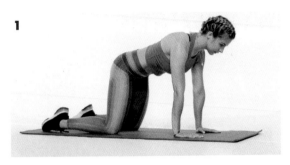

1

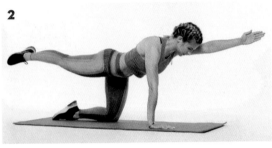

2

SETS	REPS	REST
4	5-10 reps per side	(S/S)

1 Kneel on all fours, with hands under shoulders and knees under hips. Your feet should be hip-width apart.

2 Engage your core and slowly lift and extend one arm (fingers pointed) and, at the same time, extend the opposite leg (toes pointed). Maintain a neutral spine and resist any shifts in your body weight.

3 Hold this position for 5 seconds before returning to the starting position, then repeating on the other side.

DEAD BUGS

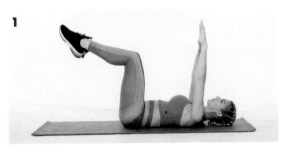

1

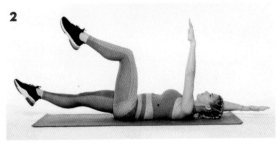

2

SETS	REPS	REST
4	5-10 reps per side	30-45 seconds

1 Lie flat on your back on the floor, with your arms extended straight out in front of you, towards the ceiling, palms facing forward. Engage your core and raise your knees into the air so they're bent at a 90-degree angle. (Basically, get into the position you would if someone said, 'be a dead beetle'!) Make sure your lower back stays flat against the floor throughout the movement.

2 Inhale and then, as you exhale, slowly lower your your right arm towards the floor behind your head, and simultaneously straighten your right leg (so it's also lowering towards the floor). Keep going until your hand and heel almost touch the floor, but stop before they do. Pause, then return to the starting position before repeating with your left arm and leg. Keep your non-moving arm and leg as stable as possible throughout this exercise.

RESISTANCE BAND ANTI-ROTATIONAL STEP BACK

SETS	REPS	REST
3	10 reps per side	(S/S)

1 Hook a resistance band over a mid-height anchor point (like a door handle). Holding the other side in both hands, with arms fully extended, stand side-on beside it, far enough away to feel tension in the band.

2 Engaging your abs, take a small step backwards with the foot furthest away from the anchor point. You should feel the glute closest to the anchor point and your obliques fire to stabilise the movement. Hold, return to the starting position and then repeat.

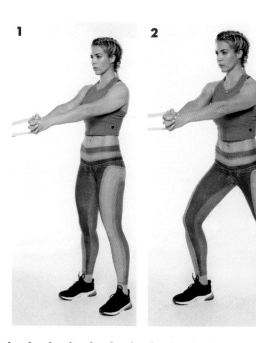

HOLLOW HOLD

SETS	REPS	REST
3	5 second hold, 5 reps	30–45 seconds

1 Lie flat on your back with your legs straight and your arms extended above your head. Engage your core.

2 Slowly raise your arms and legs at the same time so your body forms a bowl shape. (Keep your lower back on the floor; don't let it arch.) Hold this position for 5 seconds, keeping your abs tight – and remember to breathe! Return to the starting position with a controlled movement, and repeat for the desired number of reps.

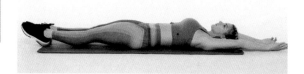

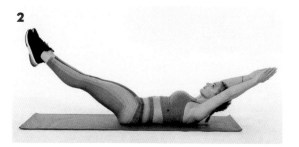

PHASE 1:

GYM STRENGTH WORKOUT

Warm-up (see page 76): **5 minutes**

Workout: **20–25 minutes**

Cool-down (see page 80): **5 minutes**

EXERCISE	SETS	REPS/TIME	REST	TARGET AREA
Dumbbell goblet bench squat	3	10–15 reps	(S/S)	Glutes, quads and hamstrings
Incline dumbbell shoulder/upper chest press	3	10–15 reps	45 seconds	Shoulders, chest and triceps
Split squats	3	10–15 reps per leg	(S/S)	Full lower body
Cable face pulls	3	8–12 reps	45 seconds	Upper back and biceps
Swiss ball leg curl	3	10–15 reps	(S/S)	Hamstrings and glutes
Triceps extension with rope attachment	3	10–15 reps	45 seconds	Triceps

DUMBBELL GOBLET BENCH SQUAT

SETS	REPS	REST
3	10–15 reps	(S/S)

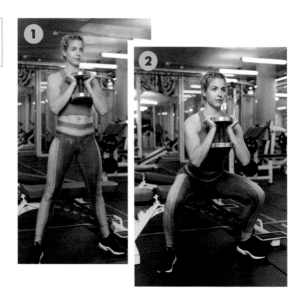

1 Stand in front of a flat bench with feet shoulder-width apart and toes slightly turned out. Using both hands, grip one dumbbell vertically (like a heavy goblet – see?) in front of your chest, with elbows tucked in.

2 Engage your core, and slowly begin to squat, sitting backwards towards the bench until your glutes just touch it. Without actually sitting, drive back up to the starting position by pushing your weight through your heels. Don't allow your knees to reach over your toes at any point. Squeeze your glutes at the top and drop your chin onto your chest to stop you from arching your lower back. Pause and repeat.

INCLINE DUMBBELL SHOULDER /UPPER CHEST PRESS

SETS	REPS	REST
3	10–15 reps	45 seconds

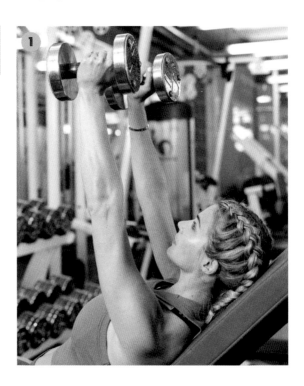

1 Set a bench to an incline of roughly 70 degrees. Sit on it and lie back with a dumbbell in each hand, palms facing each other.

2 Lift the weights so you're holding them in the air, with your arms straight, directly above your shoulders, palms still facing each other. Squeeze your shoulder blades together and create a small arch in your lower back.

3 Engaging your core, slowly lower the weights down towards your chest, stopping when you can feel a good stretch across your upper chest. Pause, then drive the weight back up to the top position. Pause again before repeating.

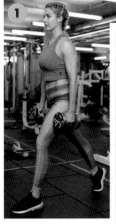

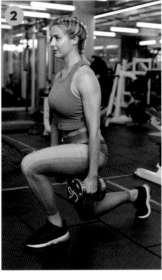

SPLIT SQUATS

SETS	REPS	REST
3	10–15 reps per leg	(S/S)

1 Standing with your feet hip-width apart, take a step forwards so your front foot is flat but your back foot is on its toes, with the heel elevated. Keep your chest up and your shoulders back, and face forwards.

2 Engage your core and slowly lower your back knee towards the floor, stopping just before you touch it. (Try not to lean too far forwards.) Pause, then drive back up through the front leg to the starting position. Repeat for the desired number of reps on one leg before alternating. To increase intensity, hold a set of dumbbells down by your sides.

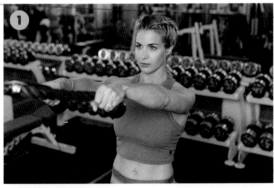

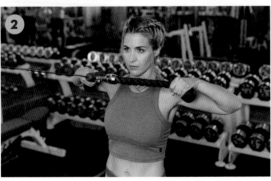

CABLE FACE PULLS

SETS	REPS	REST
3	8–12 reps	45 seconds

1 Using a cable-pulley machine, attach a rope to the high end. Stand with feet shoulder-width apart, and keep your back straight and chest proud as you hold the ends of the rope with an overhand grip.

2 Engaging your core, pull the rope directly towards your face with a controlled movement, separating your hands as you do so and keeping your upper arms parallel to the floor. Stop just short of the bridge of your nose, pause, then return to the starting position. Repeat for the desired number of reps.

SWISS BALL LEG CURL

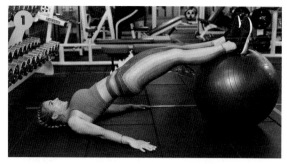

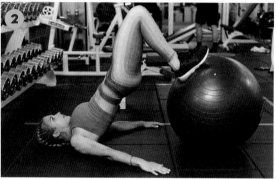

SETS	REPS	REST
3	10–15 reps	(S/S)

1 Lie on your back, with the bottom part of your legs (calves and heels) on a Swiss ball, hip-width apart. With arms by your sides and palms down, engage your core and lift your hips up towards the ceiling until your body is in a straight line.

2 From here, squeeze your glutes and slowly, with a controlled movement, bend your knees and lift your hips up even higher by pulling your heels (and rolling the ball) in towards your bum. Keep pulling until the soles of your feet are touching the ball. Hold for a second before reversing the movement. Your body should stay in the air the whole time. However, if that's too hard, you can reset from the floor position between each rep.

TRICEPS EXTENSION WITH ROPE ATTACHMENT

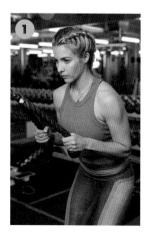

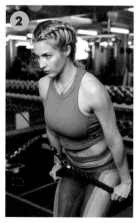

SETS	REPS	REST
3	10–15 reps	45 seconds

1 Attach a rope to the high end of a cable-pulley machine and hold it with a neutral grip, your palms facing each other. Stand with your spine straight, with a slight forward lean. Keep your upper arms close to your body, forearms bent at the elbow.

2 Engage your core and drive your hands downwards, fully extending your arms and squeezing your triceps. Don't move your upper arms or allow your elbows to flare out. Pause, then slowly return to the starting position. Repeat for the desired number of reps.

PHASE 1:

GYM CAC WORKOUT

Warm-up (see page 76): **5 minutes**

Workout: **20—25 minutes**

Cool-down (see page 80): **5 minutes**

EXERCISE	SETS	REPS/TIME	REST	TARGET AREA
KB Swings	5	20 reps	60 seconds	Hamstrings, glutes and lower back
Side plank with dumbbell rotation	5	10 reps per side	(S/S)	Obliques and core
Ab mat crunch	5	10—15 reps	45 seconds	Abs and core
Power hill walk on treadmill		10 minutes		Cardiovascular fitness

KB SWINGS

SETS	REPS	REST
5	20 reps	60 seconds

Stand with feet shoulder-width apart, with a kettlebell
between your feet. Push back with your bum, keeping
your back straight and bending your knees slightly to
get into position – like a silverback gorilla would stand!
Then, holding the kettlebell with both hands, lift it up
and gradually begin to swing it between your legs
and out in front of you. Your arms should be straight
throughout and shouldn't go higher than parallel to
the floor. Don't use your shoulders – this is a hip-hinge
movement. One back and forth (high and low) swing
counts as one rep.

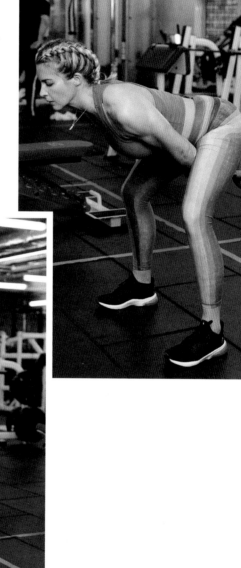

SIDE PLANK WITH DUMBBELL ROTATION

SETS	REPS	REST
5	10 reps per side	(S/S)

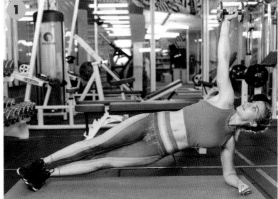

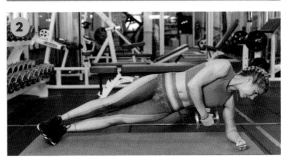

1 Lie on your right-hand side, with your right elbow positioned directly under your shoulder and hips, legs, ankles and feet stacked on top of each other. Keeping your back straight, lift your hips towards the ceiling, creating a straight line from head to toe down the centre of your body. Engage your core and squeeze your glutes, then pick up a dumbbell in your left hand before lifting your left arm straight up towards the ceiling. This is your starting position.

2 Rotate your upper body forwards and move the hand holding the dumbbell under your waist (through the gap). The arm should be kept 'long', creating a wide arc. Pause, then rotate back to the starting position, repeating for the set number of reps before swapping sides. If this is too difficult, set up as above, but keep your knees on the floor, with your legs bent at a 90-degree angle.

If you find this exercise too easy, hold a dumbbell on your chest to increase the load.

AB MAT CRUNCH

SETS	REPS	REST
5	10–15 reps	45 seconds

1 Lie flat with an ab mat resting in the natural arch of your lower back (you can also use a rolled-up towel or folded floor mat). Bend your knees at a 45-degree angle, with feet flat on the floor. Rest your hands on the sides of your thighs.

2 Engage your core and slowly lift your upper body towards the ceiling, trying to flatten your lower back into the ab mat. Only rise a few inches off the floor. As you do so, run your hands up your thighs. Exhale at the top and contract your abs for a second before slowly lowering yourself back to the starting position to repeat. Rest your head on the floor between reps.

POWER HILL WALK ON TREADMILL

TIME
10 minutes

Set the gradient on a treadmill to 4–8%. Select a
speed of 5–6 kmph, depending on your fitness level.
You'll be doing 10 minutes, working at 50–65% of
your max heart rate. You should be sweating slightly
but not be too out of breath: it should be a brisk walk.
Make sure to maintain your body posture, and
don't hold onto the bar in front of you.

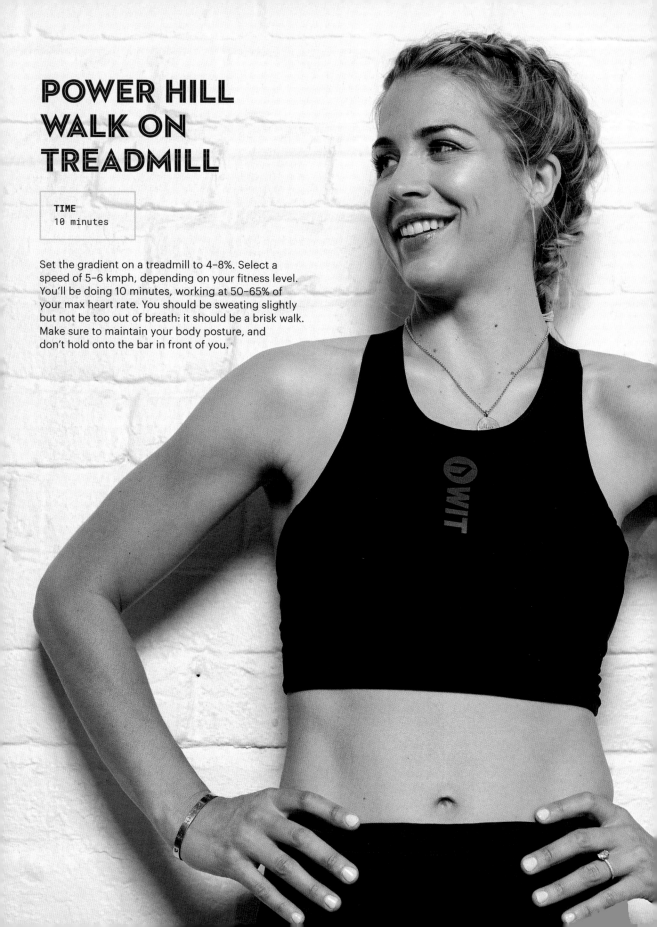

PHASE 2:

HOME STRENGTH WORKOUT

Warm-up (see page 76): **5 minutes**

Workout: **20–25 minutes**

Cool-down (see page 80): **5 minutes**

EXERCISE	SETS	REPS/TIME	REST	TARGET AREA
Elevated glute bridge – body weight only	3	10–15 reps	(S/S)	Glute and hamstring activation
Resistance band RDL	3	10–15 reps	45 seconds	Glutes and hamstrings
Straight arm resistance band pull-downs	3	10–15 reps	(S/S)	Chest and lats
Resistance band side lateral raises	3	10–15 reps	45 seconds	Shoulders
Single-leg chair pistol squats	3	10–15 reps per leg	(S/S)	Glutes, hamstring and quads
Chair dips	3	10–15 reps	45 seconds	Triceps

ELEVATED GLUTE BRIDGE (body weight only)

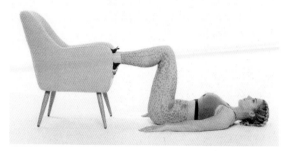

1

SETS	REPS	REST
3	10–15 reps	(S/S)

1 Lie on your back with the bottom half of your legs resting on the seat of a chair (knees bent at a 90-degree angle) and your arms resting by your sides on the floor.

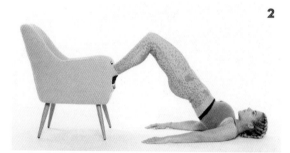

2

2 Engage your core and drive your hips up into the air, pushing down through your heels. Take your hips as far up as you can without arching your lower back. Squeeze your bum cheeks together at the top by tucking your pelvis 'in and under'. Reverse the movement, with control, and repeat.

//

RESISTANCE BAND RDL

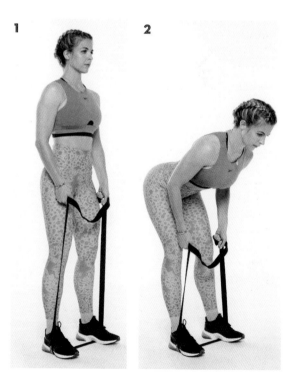

SETS	REPS	REST
3	10–15 reps	45 seconds

1 Stand on the middle of a resistance band with your feet hip-width apart. Grab the other side of the band in your hands, with a slight bend in your knees.

2 Engaging your core and keeping your knees slightly flexed, slowly lower your face towards the floor by hinging your hips, keeping your back straight. Your hamstrings should stretch. Pause here for a second, then, without arching or rounding your back, bring yourself back up to the starting position (you shouldn't be 'pulling' the band with your biceps). Squeeze your glutes at the top by tucking your pelvis in and dropping your chin to your chest. Hold for a second, then repeat for the desired number of reps.

STRAIGHT ARM RESISTANCE BAND PULL-DOWNS

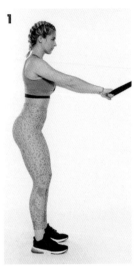
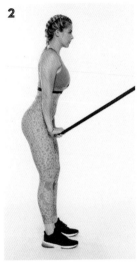

SETS	REPS	REST
3	10–15 reps	(S/S)

1 Attach your resistance band to an anchor point at or just above head height. Facing the anchor point, grip the other side of the band in both hands, palms facing each other, and step back until your arms are fully extended and you can feel tension in the band. Bend your hips back slightly so your upper body is at about a 45-degree angle, and drop your shoulders down.

2 Keeping your arms straight, pull them down slowly to your sides in an arching motion so your hands end up in line with your hips. Pause here for a second before slowly returning to the starting position, then repeat.

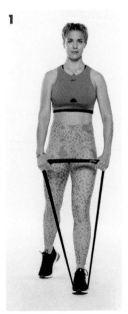
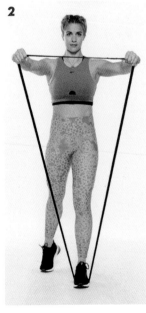

RESISTANCE BAND SIDE LATERAL RAISES

SETS	REPS	REST
3	10–15 reps	45 seconds

1 Get into a split stance position with your left foot in front and in the middle of a resistance band. Grab the other side of the band with an overhand grip, palms facing towards you.

2 With shoulder blades back and chest up, engage your core and, without swinging, raise your arms to shoulder-height, keeping a slight bend in the elbows. Don't arch your lower back. Pause, then slowly lower back to the starting position and repeat.

SINGLE-LEG CHAIR PISTOL SQUATS

SETS	REPS	REST
3	10–15 reps per leg	(S/S)

1 Stand in front of a chair on one foot, the other hovering just off the floor. Keep your weight in the heel of your fixed leg, core engaged.

2 Pushing your hips backwards and bending the knee of your fixed leg, lower yourself into a seated position. (The leg floating in the air shouldn't touch the ground at all.) Tap your bum on the chair, then immediately push yourself back up to a standing position. Repeat.

* If this is too hard, add some pillows to the chair to reduce the distance. If it's too easy, hold a water bottle at chest height, keeping your elbows tucked in.

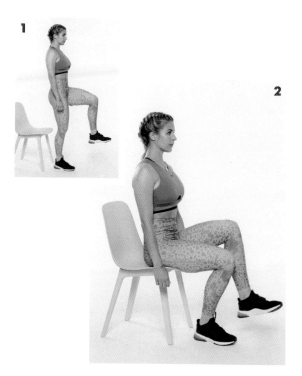

CHAIR DIPS

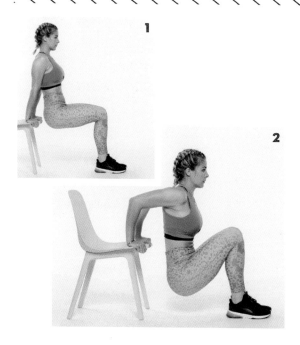

SETS	REPS	REST
3	10–15 reps	45 seconds

1 Sit on the edge of a chair with your hands gripping the sides of the seat. Lift your bum off the seat and walk your feet slightly forwards, knees bent at a 90-degree angle, upper body straight.

2 Engage your core and slowly lower your bum towards the floor, with your hands still gripping the chair. Once your elbows are bent at a 90-degree angle, stop. Hold this position for a second before driving your body weight back up by straightening your arms. Make sure your body doesn't slide forwards – aim to keep your bum as close to the chair edge as possible without actually touching it. Repeat for the desired number of reps.

PHASE 2:

HOME CAC WORKOUT

Warm-up (see page 76): **5 minutes**

Workout: **20–25 minutes**

Cool-down (see page 80): **5 minutes**

EXERCISE	SETS	REPS/TIME	REST	TARGET AREA
Step downs	5	10–15 reps per side	(S/S)	Lower body
High plank with outside knee tuck	5	5–10 reps per side	45–60 seconds	Abs, core and hips
Lateral hops	4	20–30 reps	(S/S)	Lower body
Side plank with rotation	4	5 reps per side	45–60 seconds	Obliques and core
Lying oblique twists	3	5 reps per side	(S/S)	Obliques and core
Reverse crunch	3	10–15 reps	45 seconds	Abs and core

STEP DOWNS

SETS	REPS	REST
5	10–15 reps per side	(S/S)

1 Stand with feet hip-width apart, chest puffed out and core engaged.

2 'Step down' with your right leg until your knee touches the floor and then 'step down' with your left leg until you are in a kneeling position. Pause, and then lift your right leg up, placing the foot squarely down on the floor so you can drive yourself back up to standing position. Complete the desired number of reps on one side before swapping to the other.

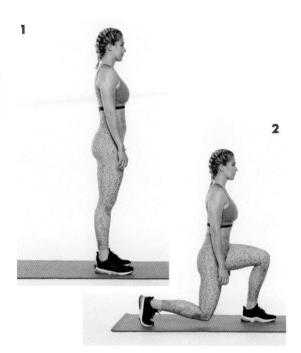

HIGH PLANK WITH OUTSIDE KNEE TUCK

SETS	REPS	REST
5	5–10 reps per side	45–60 seconds

1 Get into a push-up position on the floor with your core engaged.

2 Making sure your body is in a straight line parallel to the floor, bring your right leg out to the side and try to touch your right elbow with your knee (you don't have to actually touch the elbow, but that's the direction you should make the movement in). Return your leg to the starting position and repeat on the other side. Keep alternating legs, aiming for 5–10 reps per side.

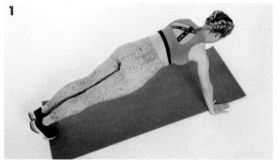

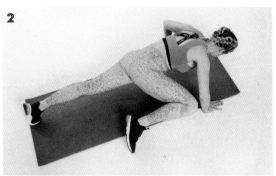

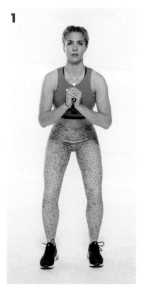
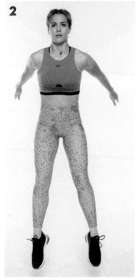

LATERAL HOPS

SETS	REPS	REST
4	20–30 reps	(S/S)

Stand tall with feet hip-width apart and knees soft. Jump from side-to-side with both legs, as if you're jumping over a small obstacle. Make sure to land with soft knees, trying to remain on the balls of your feet.

SIDE PLANK
WITH ROTATION

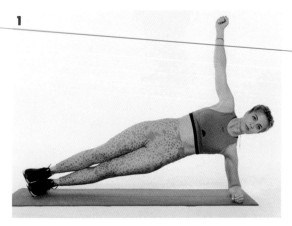
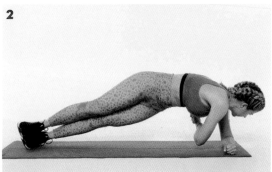

SETS	REPS	REST
4	5 reps per side	45–60 seconds

1 Lie on your left-hand side, with your left elbow positioned directly under your shoulder and your hips, legs, ankles and feet stacked on top of each other. Keeping your back straight and your head in a neutral position, lift your hips towards the ceiling, creating a straight line from head to toe down the centre of your body. Engage your core and squeeze your glutes before lifting your right arm straight up towards the ceiling. This is your starting position.

2 Rotate your upper body forwards and reach under your waist with your right arm (through the gap) as if you're trying to touch something behind you. The arm should be kept 'long', creating a wide arc. Pause, then rotate back to the starting position, repeating for the set number of reps before swapping sides. If this is too difficult, perform as above, but keep your knees on the floor.

LYING OBLIQUE TWISTS

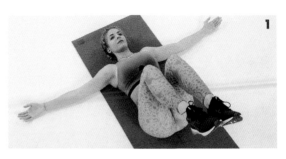

SETS	REPS	REST
3	5 reps side	(S/S)

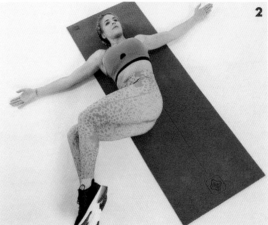

1 Lie on your back and place your arms out to the side in a T-shape, with your palms facing upwards. Engage your core and lift your legs up into the air so they're bent at a 90-degree angle and your ankles are in line with your knees. Keep your lower back flat on the floor. This is your starting position.

2 Keeping ankles and knees pressed together, slowly lower your legs down towards the right, by rotating the hips, until they nearly touch the floor. Pause, then return your legs to the starting position before repeating on the other side. Your upper body should remain stable and fixed to the floor throughout the whole movement. To make this exercise more difficult, extend your leg length, keeping your ankles and feet together, and go high to create a wider arc.

REVERSE CRUNCH

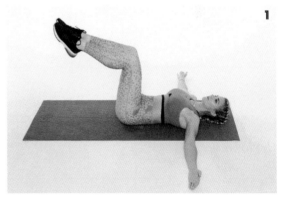

SETS	REPS	REST
3	10–15 reps	45 seconds

1 Lie on your back with your arms in a T-shape, palms facing up. Your legs should be raised, your thighs vertical and your knees bent at a 90-degree angle.

2 With your core engaged and knees bent throughout, slowly lower your feet towards the ground until you feel a slight arch in your lower back. When your heels are nearly touching the ground, use your abs to bring your knees back up towards the chest, flattening your lower back into the ground. Hold for a second before slowly lowering the legs back down to repeat for the desired number of reps. Your legs shouldn't flex or extend throughout this movement.

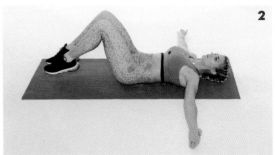

PHASE 2:

GYM STRENGTH WORKOUT

Warm-up (see page 76): **5 minutes**

Workout: **20–25 minutes**

Cool-down (see page 80): **5 minutes**

EXERCISE	SETS	REPS/TIME	REST	TARGET AREA
Cable rope pull-through	3	10–15 reps	(S/S)	Glutes, hip flexors, hamstrings and lower back
Cable rope straight arm pull-downs	3	10–15 reps	45 seconds	Lats and chest
Single-leg leg press	3	10–15 reps per leg	(S/S)	Glutes, hamstrings and quads
Swiss ball dumbbell lateral raises	3	10–15 reps	45 seconds	Shoulders and core
Barbell glute bridge	3	10–15 reps	(S/S)	Glutes and hamstrings
Swiss ball triceps extension	3	10–15 reps	45 seconds	Triceps and core

CABLE ROPE PULL-THROUGH

SETS	REPS	REST
3	10–15 reps	(S/S)

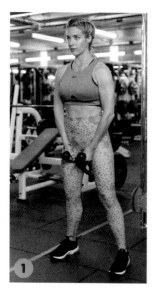

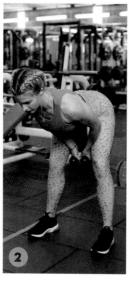

1 Attach a rope to the cable machine at the lowest setting. Facing away from the machine, stand with the rope attachment between your legs, then pick it up with your palms facing together. Step forwards until the weight stack lifts – it should remain lifted throughout the movement. Set your feet roughly shoulder-width apart, with shoulders back and down, chest up, head neutral and core engaged.

2 Begin the movement by pushing your hips back towards the machine, without losing spine alignment, until you feel a stretch in your hamstrings. (Your arms follow the movement as 'bossed' by the hips – they don't dictate the move.) Pause, then reverse by driving your hips forwards until you're back in the starting position. Here, tuck your pelvis in and drop your chin while squeezing the glutes. Repeat for the desired number of reps.

CABLE ROPE STRAIGHT ARM PULL-DOWNS

SETS	REPS	REST
3	10–15 reps	45 seconds

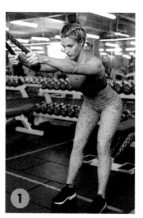

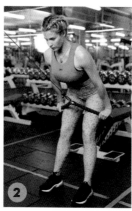

1 This time, reattach the rope on the cable at the top setting. Facing this anchor point, hold the rope with your palms facing inwards and take a few steps back to lift the weight off the stack. Bend your hips back slightly so your upper body is at a roughly 45-degree angle, with your arms straight and a soft flex in your knees. This is your starting position.

2 You should already feel a slight stretch in your lats. Now, keeping your elbows locked, drive your arms slowly down to your sides in a smooth motion so your hands end up just behind your hips. Pause here for a second before slowly returning to the starting position and repeat.

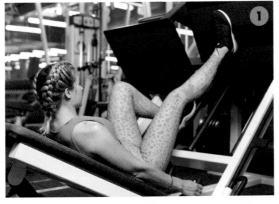

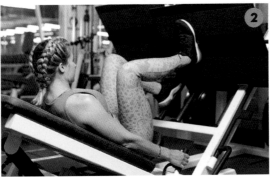

SINGLE-LEG LEG PRESS

SETS	REPS	REST
3	10–15 reps per leg	(S/S)

1 Position yourself on a leg-press machine with your feet hip-width apart and slightly higher than the midline of the foot plate. Select a light weight to begin with and, with your core engaged, push the plate away with both legs to almost full knee extension (make sure you don't lock your knees – they must have a slight flex in them at all times). Unhook the safety latch, then remove one foot from the plate. This is your starting position.

2 Making sure your core is still engaged, lower the weight until your knee is bent at or just past 90 degrees and tracks over the toe line. Pause here for a second, then drive your leg away, pushing through the heel of your working leg, stopping just short of lockout. Repeat for the desired number of reps before swapping legs.

SWISS BALL DUMBBELL LATERAL RAISES

SETS	REPS	REST
3	10–15 reps per leg	45 seconds

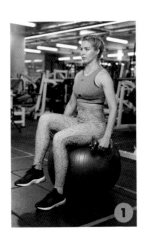
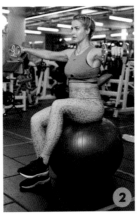

1 Sit upright on a Swiss ball, with your chest up and your shoulders back and down. Hold a pair of dumbbells down by your sides. This is your starting position.

2 With your core engaged, laterally lift your arms up to shoulder height with a slight bend in the elbows and your palms facing towards the floor. Hold for a second, before slowly returning to the starting position with a controlled movement. Repeat for the desired number of reps. To challenge your core further, you can do the same exercise with only one foot placed on the floor and the other slightly lifted. This will create less stability and require your core to work harder to maintain your posture.

BARBELL GLUTE BRIDGE

SETS	REPS	REST
3	10–15 reps	(S/S)

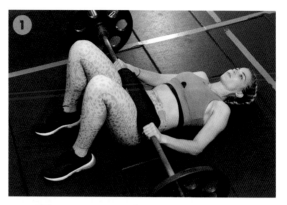

1 Sit on the floor and roll a loaded barbell over your legs until it's sitting directly above your hips (if the bar hurts when you lift up your hips, wrap your towel around it or put a pad between it and your body). Lie down so you're flat on your back, and bring your feet up towards your bum so your knees are at a 45-degree angle. This is your starting position.

2 Holding the bar steady with extended arms, thrust your hips up towards the ceiling as far as possible, lifting the barbell with them. Push your weight through your heels and keep your upper back, neck and head on the ground. Squeeze your glutes at the top without arching your lower back, then slowly return back to the starting position before pausing and repeating.

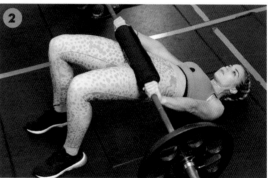

SWISS BALL TRICEPS EXTENSION

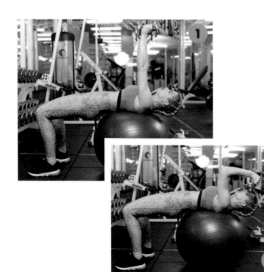

SETS	REPS	REST
3	10–15 reps	45 seconds

1 Sit upright on a Swiss ball holding a set of dumbbells on your thighs. Engage your core and walk your feet forwards until your middle and upper back are supported by the ball. Set your knees at a 90-degree angle, feet planted. Holding the dumbbells, extend your arms above you with your palms facing inwards. Lift your hips until your body is in a straight line from head to knees.

2 Slowly lower the dumbbells by bending your arms at the elbows. Make sure your upper arms don't move. Stop when the dumbbells touch the front of your shoulders. Hold for a second, then return to the starting position with a controlled movement.

PHASE 2:

GYM CAC WORKOUT

Warm-up (see page 76): **5 minutes**

Workout: **20–25 minutes**

Cool-down (see page 80): **5 minutes**

EXERCISE	SETS	REPS/TIME	REST	TARGET AREA
Rower warm-up		3 minutes		Cardiovascular fitness
Rower	5–10	30 seconds	60 seconds	Anaerobic fitness
Rower cool-down		3 minutes		Cardiovascular fitness
Russian twist with medicine ball	3	10 reps per side	45 seconds	Obliques and core
Hanging leg raise with legs bent	3	10–15 reps	(S/S)	Abs and core
Hanging leg raise with legs straight	3	10–15 reps	45 seconds	Abs and core

ROWER

SETS	TIME
1	3 minutes

Using the rowing machine, row for 3 minutes at about 50–60% of your maximum effort rate, to the point where you build up a slight sweat. This is a mini warm-up for the rowing exercise ahead (you should still complete the official warm-up on page 76 before starting this session).

SETS	TIME
5–10	30 seconds

Maintaining good form, now row as fast as you comfortably can, at 70–85% of your maximum effort rate, for 30 seconds. Then rest, by either stopping completely or by rowing slowly for 60 seconds. This is considered 1 interval or set. Repeat for a further 4 sets. If you have time, and really want to challenge yourself, increase the amount of sets you do – but don't do more than 10.

SETS	TIME	REST
1	3 minutes	Cool down

Do exactly the same as you did for your rowing warm-up to cool down: 3 minutes at 50–60% effort. (Again, you should still complete the official cool-down on page 80 when you reach the end of the session.)

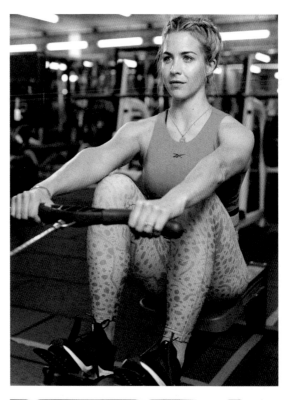

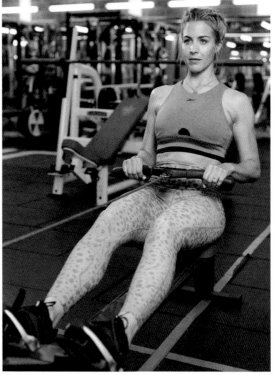

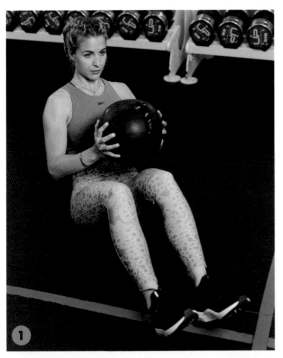

RUSSIAN TWIST WITH MEDICINE BALL

SETS	REPS	REST
3	10 reps per side	45 seconds

1 Sit on the mat with your back straight, knees bent and heels resting on the floor. Hold a medicine ball just in front of your chest with both hands, with your elbows bent. Lean back slightly until you feel your core working.

2 In a slow, controlled movement, twist your upper body to the left. Hold this position for a moment, then return to centre before twisting to the right. Continue for the desired number of reps.

This exercise is not recommended if you have any problems with your lower back. It's also important that you pay close attention to your form to prevent injury.

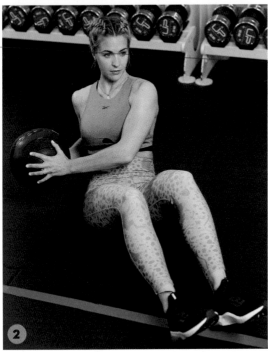

HANGING LEG RAISE WITH LEGS BENT

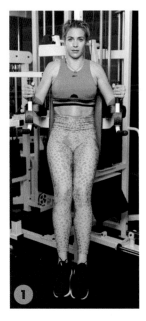
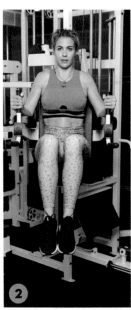

SETS	REPS	REST
3	10–15 reps	(S/S)

1 Stand with your back to the 'Captain's chair' or 'Roman chair'. Place your arms on the arm rests and grip the handles firmly. With control, lift your body up until you are in the position shown in image 1.

2 Slowly and with control, lift your legs, drawing your knees up towards your chest until they reach a 90-degree angle. Hold for a moment, then slowly lower to repeat the movement.

HANGING LEG RAISE WITH LEGS STRAIGHT

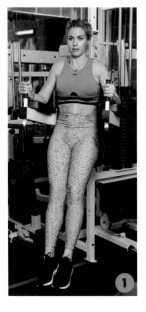
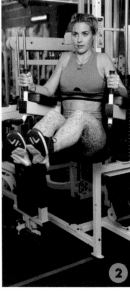

SETS	REPS	REST
3	10–15 reps	45 seconds

1 Staying in the 'Captain's chair', get into the same position as in the previous exercise: body and legs straight, feet lifted off the floor.

2 This time, keep your legs straight (with a soft bend in the knees). Slowly and with control, lift your legs out in front of you. Hold, then lower slowly before repeating.

PHASE 3:
HOME STRENGTH WORKOUT

Warm-up (see page 76): **5 minutes**

Workout: **20—25 minutes**

Cool-down (see page 80): **5 minutes**

EXERCISE	SETS	REPS/TIME	REST	TARGET AREA
Resistance band front squat into shoulder press	3	10—15 reps	45 seconds	Shoulders and lower body
Resistance band seated row	3	10—15 reps	45 seconds	Back and biceps
Resistance band single-leg RDL	3	10—15 reps per leg	(S/S)	Glutes, hip flexors, hamstrings and lower back
Resistance band lateral lunge	3	10—15 reps per leg	(S/S)	Lower body (inc. adductors)
Body weight push-ups	3	10—15 reps	45 seconds	Chest and triceps

RESISTANCE BAND FRONT SQUAT INTO SHOULDER PRESS

SETS	REPS	REST
3	10–15 reps	45 seconds

1 Stand on the middle of a resistance band with feet hip-width apart. Hold the other side of the band in your hands, with palms facing upwards and arms fully extended into the air. Keep your back straight, your chest up, your head forward and your core engaged. This is your starting position.

2 Squat down towards the ground by pushing your hips backwards and bending at the knees, allowing them to track forwards slightly – think silverback gorilla. At the point where your thighs are parallel to the floor, pause, then drive your hips back up to the starting position, while simultaneously pushing your arms straight up towards the ceiling (don't rotate the palms). Pause at the top and then repeat.

* If you feel like your squat depth is poor, try elevating your heels by resting them on a book.

1

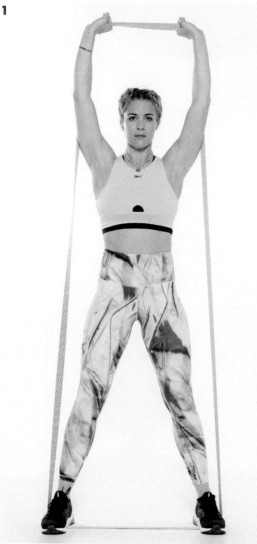

2

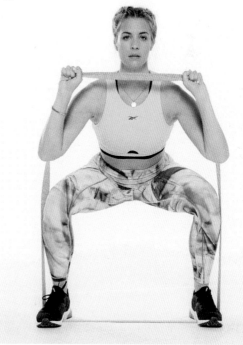

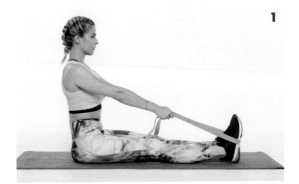

RESISTANCE BAND SEATED ROW

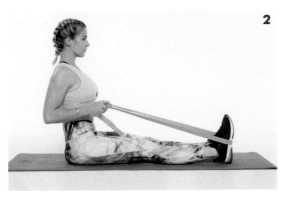

SETS	REPS	REST
3	10–15 reps	45 seconds

1 Sit on the floor and extend your legs out in front of you with a slight bend in your knees, keeping your upper body tall and your chest high. Wrap the middle of the resistance band around your feet, holding the other side at arm's length, with palms facing inwards.

2 Engage your core and pull the band towards you by squeezing your shoulder blades and pulling your elbows back. Don't let your wrists flex, and make sure to keep your elbows tight to the sides of your body. Hold for a second here, then reverse the movement, moving with control, before repeating.

RESISTANCE BAND SINGLE-LEG RDL

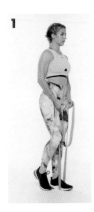
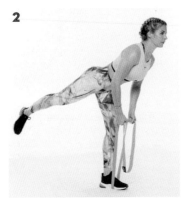

SETS	REPS	REST
3	10–15 reps per leg	(S/S)

1 Stand on the middle of your resistance band with one foot, gripping the other end in both hands, palms facing each other. Lift your other foot into the air.

2 Engage your core and, flexing at the hips, start to lean forwards while simultaneously taking your lifted leg backwards as a counterbalance, keeping it relatively straight. Keep moving until your torso is parallel to the floor, making sure you don't arch your lower back. You should feel a good stretch in your hamstring. Pause here, then bring yourself back up to the starting position, where you should feel the tension in the band kick in. If you don't, move your grip lower down the band (closer to the floor). Try not to touch the floor with your non-working leg between reps.

RESISTANCE BAND LATERAL LUNGE

SETS	REPS	REST
3	10–15 reps per leg	(S/S)

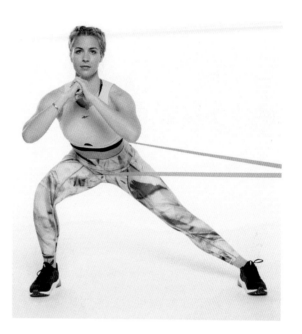

1 Attach a closed resistance band to a low anchor point and step inside it so the band is looped around your hips. Stand side-on to the anchor point, then take a few side steps away. Engage your core and, with a straight back, lean forwards slightly and flex your knees. This is your starting position.

2 Take a big step away from the anchor point with your outside foot, keeping your other foot where it is. Lower yourself down into a squat over the outside foot while keeping your trailing leg straight. Drive back up to the starting position. Repeat on the same leg for the desired number of reps before swapping.

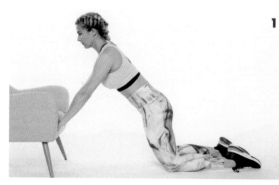

1

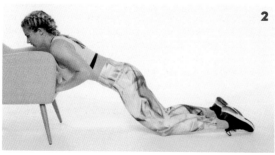

2

BODY-WEIGHT PUSH-UPS

SETS	REPS	REST
3	10–15 reps	45 seconds

1 Kneeling on the floor, place your hands shoulder-width apart on the edge of a chair or sofa seat. Keeping your back straight and your pelvis neutral, engage your core. Don't arch your lower back.

2 Slowly lower your torso towards the chair by bending your elbows (they should be at about a 45-degree angle to your body). Stop just before your chest touches the chair. Hold for a second before driving back to the starting position, making sure not to round your upper back.

PHASE 3:

HOME CAC WORKOUT

Warm-up (see page 76): **5 minutes**

Workout: **20–25 minutes**

Cool-down (see page 80): **5 minutes**

EXERCISE	SETS	REPS/TIME	REST	TARGET AREA
Tuck jumps	5	10–15 reps	(S/S)	Lower body
High plank with inside knee tuck	5	10 reps per side	45-60 seconds	Core, abs and obliques
Side plank with top leg elevation	4	10 reps per side	45-60 seconds	Abs, core, obliques and glutes
Torso-rotation reverse lunge	4	10–15 reps per side	(S/S)	Lower body/torso mobility
Plank step-ups	3	30 seconds	(S/S)	Core, chest, triceps and shoulders
Overhead full sit-ups	3	10–15 reps	45-60 seconds	Abs and core

TUCK JUMPS

SETS	REPS	REST
5	10–15 reps	S/S

Stand with your feet hip-width apart and your arms by your sides. Perform a small squat to load your weight into the ground. From there, jump up into the air as high as you can, bringing your knees up towards your chest (like you're 'bombing' in a swimming pool) and using your arms to gain power. Ensure a good soft landing by bending your knees slightly upon impact before repeating for the set number of reps.

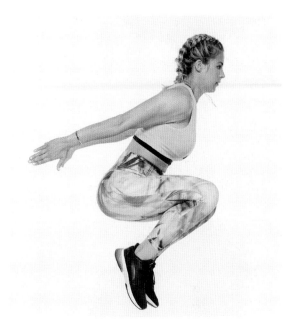

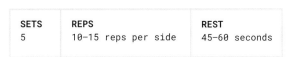

HIGH PLANK WITH INSIDE KNEE TUCK

SETS	REPS	REST
5	10–15 reps per side	45–60 seconds

1

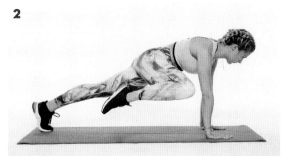

2

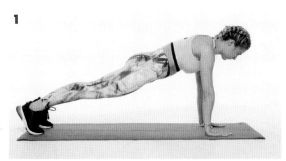

1 Hold yourself in a full push-up position on the floor, with your core engaged. Make sure your body is in a straight line parallel to the floor.

2 Tuck your right knee under your body, aiming it towards your left elbow. Return your leg to the starting position and repeat on alternate legs.

SIDE PLANK WITH TOP LEG ELEVATION

SETS	REPS	REST
4	10 reps per side	45–60 seconds

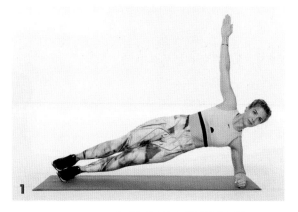

1 Lie on your left-hand side, propping yourself up on your left elbow, which should be positioned directly underneath your shoulder. Your hips, legs, ankles and feet should be stacked on top of each other. Lift your hips towards the ceiling to create a straight line from head to toe down the centre of your body. Engage your core, squeeze your glutes, and lift your right arm straight towards the ceiling.

2 Next, lift your right leg into the air as well, as high as possible. Repeat before swapping sides. If this is too difficult, keep your bottom leg on the floor and bend your knees at a 90-degree angle.

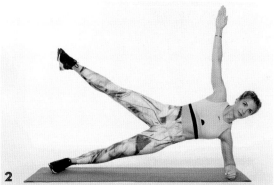

TORSO-ROTATION REVERSE LUNGE

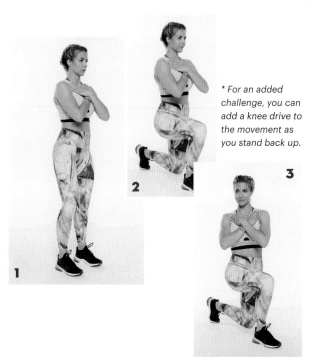

For an added challenge, you can add a knee drive to the movement as you stand back up.

SETS	REPS	REST
4	10–15 reps per side	(S/S)

1 Stand tall with feet hip-width apart, chest up, shoulders back and down, core engage and arms crossed over your chest.

2 Step back with your left leg and slowly lower your left knee towards the ground, loading your weight into your right leg and bending your right knee.

3 When your left knee is just shy of the floor, lean your upper body forwards slightly and rotate your torso to the right as far as you comfortably can without losing posture. Return your shoulders to a square position and drive yourself back up to standing. Repeat this whole movement for the desired number of reps before alternating legs.

PLANK STEP-UPS

SETS	REPS	REST
3	30 seconds	(S/S)

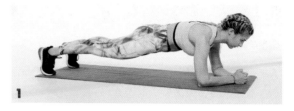

1 Get into a forearm plank position, supporting your weight through your forearms and toes. Make sure your elbows sit directly below your shoulder joints. Lift your hips up so your pelvis is in a neutral position and hold, squeezing your glutes and keeping your abs tight.

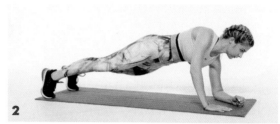

2 Lift your body into a push-up position by stepping up each arm individually.

3 Once there, step back down into the plank position again, then continue this up and down movement for the set amount of time.

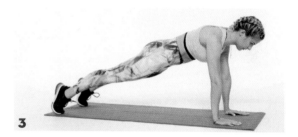

OVERHEAD FULL SIT-UPS

SETS	REPS	REST
3	10–15 reps	45–60 seconds

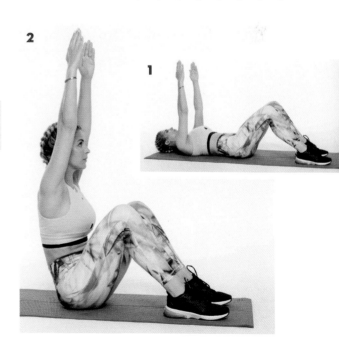

1 Lie on your back with knees and ankles together, knees bent at a 45-degree angle. Extend your arms towards the ceiling, palms facing each other.

2 Keeping your arms vertical, perform a full sit-up, raising your upper body to an upright position using only your abs. When you reach the top of the movement, both your upper body and arms should be vertical (i.e. pointing towards the ceiling). Pause and, with a controlled movement, lower yourself back down to the starting position. Repeat for the desired number of reps.

PHASE 3:

GYM STRENGTH WORKOUT

Warm-up (see page 76): **5 minutes**

Workout: **20–25 minutes**

Cool-down (see page 80): **5 minutes**

EXERCISE	SETS	REPS/TIME	REST	TARGET AREA
Dumbbell single-leg RDL	3	10–15 reps per leg	(S/S)	Glutes, hamstrings, core and stability
Dumbbell single-arm single-leg rotating shoulder press	3	10–15 reps per side	45 seconds	Shoulders, triceps, core and stability
Wide stance box squats	3	10–15 reps	(S/S)	Glutes, hamstrings and quads
Incline dumbbell prone row	3	10–15 reps	45 seconds	Back and biceps
Dumbbell walking lunges (long strides)	3	10–15 reps per leg	(S/S)	Glutes, hamstrings and quads
Swiss ball dumbbell close-grip chest press	3	10–15 reps	45 seconds	Chest, triceps and core

DUMBBELL SINGLE-LEG RDL

SETS	REPS	REST
3	10–15 reps per leg	(S/S)

1 Hold a dumbbell in each hand, with your arms hanging neutrally by your sides. Lift your right heel slightly off the ground and find your balance.

2 Bend your left knee slightly and extend your right leg backwards as a counterbalance as you lower your torso towards the floor. Your arms should remain hanging loose and your back should stay flat. Stop when your torso is parallel with the floor, pause for one second, then drive your weight through the heel of your left foot and return to the starting position, tucking your pelvis in and under to squeeze your glutes. Repeat for the desired number of reps before swapping legs. If this is too hard, only hold one dumbbell (holding the dumbbell on the same side as the swinging leg).

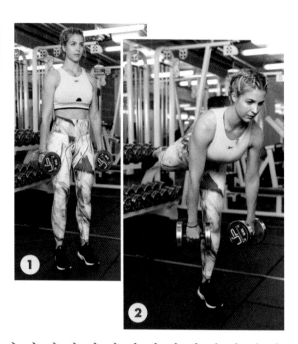

DUMBBELL SINGLE-ARM SINGLE-LEG ROTATING SHOULDER PRESS

SETS	REPS	REST
3	10–15 reps per side	45 seconds

1 Holding a dumbbell in your right hand, lift it up to shoulder height with your palm facing inwards. Lift your left leg so your thigh is parallel with the floor, knee bent at a 90-degree angle, and stretch out your left arm for balance.

2 Press your dumbbell up towards the ceiling, rotating your forearm and palm clockwise, and extending your arm fully with the weight directly above your shoulder at all times. Your palm should now be facing away from you. Pause at the top. Slowly reverse the movement until you're back in the starting position, keeping your leg lifted. Repeat for the desired number of reps before changing sides.

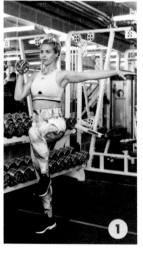
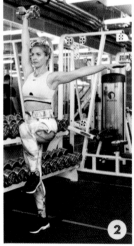

WIDE STANCE BOX SQUATS

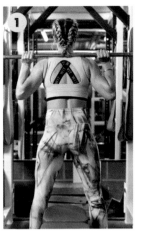
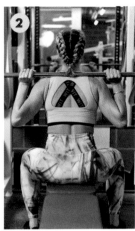

SETS	REPS	REST
3	10–15 reps	(S/S)

1 Set up a barbell in the squat rack with your chosen weight, with the bar at collarbone height. Place a bench about 3 steps behind you. Step under the barbell so that it rests across the back of your shoulders. Hold with a wide overhand grip. Stand up straight so the bar lifts off the rack. Step back until you're about a foot in front of the bench. Position your feet just wider than shoulder-width apart, toes slightly pointed out. Engage your core.

2 Slowly, with control, sit backwards towards the bench by pushing your hips and bum backwards and bending your knees. DON'T let your knees collapse inwards. Sit on the bench and pause for a second, then drive yourself back up to standing, keeping your upper body tall. Squeeze your glutes, pause, then repeat for the desired number of reps.

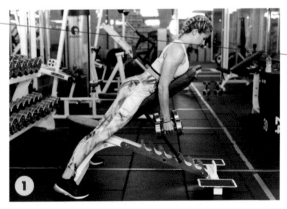

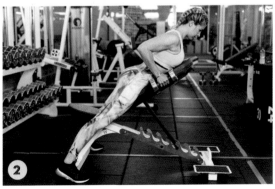

INCLINE DUMBBELL PRONE ROW

SETS	REPS	REST
3	10–15 reps	45 seconds

1 Set a bench to a 45-degree angle and lie with your chest on it, with your head sticking out over the top. Your legs should be shoulder-width apart for good stability. Holding a set of dumbbells, let your arms hang naturally down by your sides.

2 Keeping your head up and abs engaged, slowly bring your shoulder blades together, pulling the weights towards your chest by driving your elbows back towards the ceiling. Pause at your top end range, without bending your wrists, then slowly lower the weights back down to the starting position. Repeat.

DUMBBELL WALKING LUNGES (LONG STRIDES)

SETS	REPS	REST
3	10–15 reps per leg	(S/S)

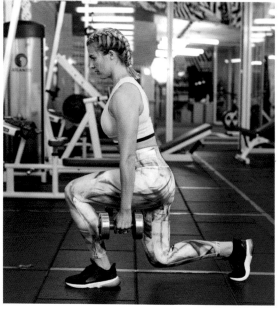

1 Stand straight with your feet shoulder-width apart. Hold a set of dumbbells in your hands, arms by your sides, palms facing inwards. Take a big step forwards, planting your front foot heel first. With control, bend both knees until your back knee is just shy of the floor. Your front knee should track over the toe line. Pause, keeping most of your weight in your front leg.

2 Stand up by driving your weight through your front heel, bringing your back foot to meet the front foot. Repeat with opposing legs for the desired number of reps so you're 'walking' forwards.

SWISS BALL DUMBBELL CLOSE-GRIP CHEST PRESS

SETS	REPS	REST
3	10–15 reps	45 seconds

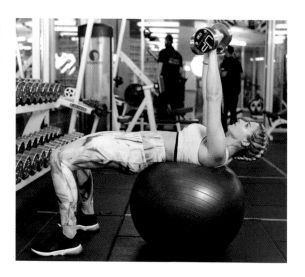

1 Sit on a Swiss ball, holding a set of dumbbells. Walk your feet forwards until your middle and upper back are supported by the ball. Set your knees at a 90-degree angle, feet planted.

2 Extend your arms upwards with your palms facing inwards. Lift your hips so they are in line with your torso (there should be a slight arch in your lower back). Engage your core.

3 With control, lower the dumbbells towards your chest until you feel a deep stretch. Pause, then drive them back upwards by extending your arms. Repeat for the desired number of reps.

PHASE 3:

GYM CAC WORKOUT

Warm-up (see page 76): **5 minutes**

Workout: **20–25 minutes**

Cool-down (see page 80): **5 minutes**

EXERCISE	SETS	REPS/TIME	REST	TARGET AREA
Body-weight box jumps	4	15–20 reps	(S/S)	Lower body
Overhead medicine-ball slams or rope slams	4	15–20 reps	60–75 seconds	Upper body
Swiss ball knee tucks	3	10–15 reps	(S/S)	Abs and core
Swiss ball plank (with 'stirring the pot')	3	20–30 seconds	30–45 seconds	Abs and core
Airdyne bike	5	60 seconds	60 seconds	Cardiovascular fitness

BODY-WEIGHT BOX JUMPS

SETS	REPS	REST
4	15–20 reps	(S/S)

1 Grab a jump box – I'd recommend starting with a box that's roughly mid-shin height, and aiming to progress to knee-height or slightly above during the four weeks. Stand in front of it with feet hip-width apart and arms by your sides.

2 Perform a small squat to load your weight into the ground, then jump up and forwards into the air as high as you can, bringing your knees up to your chest and using your arms to increase power. Ensure a good soft landing on the box by bending the knees slightly upon impact.

3 Stand up straight, then step backwards off the box before repeating for the desired number of reps.

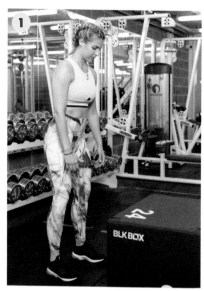

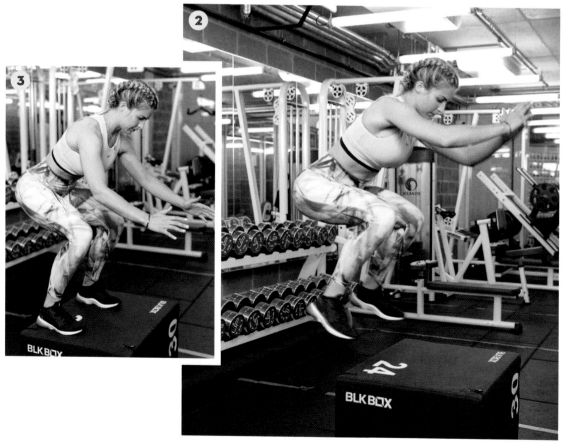

OVERHEAD MEDICINE-BALL SLAMS OR ROPE SLAMS

SETS	REPS	REST
4	15–20 reps	60–75 seconds

1 Hold a medicine ball with both hands at waist height. Stand on tiptoes with your feet shoulder-width apart. Start the movement by raising the ball above your head, fully extending your arms.

2 From this top position, slam the ball down into the ground in front of you as hard as possible. Retrieve the ball and repeat this movement for the desired number of reps. (If your gym doesn't have a medicine ball, you can use warrior ropes. Start by holding the ropes at hip height, then lift them up to shoulder height before driving them back towards the ground.)

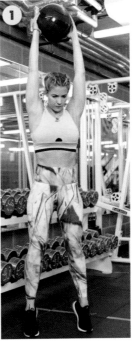
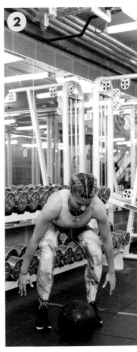

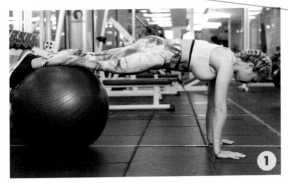
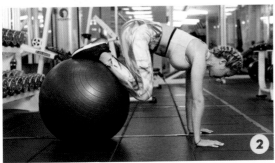

SWISS BALL KNEE TUCKS

SETS	REPS	REST
3	10–15 reps	(S/S)

1 Kneeling behind a Swiss ball, roll yourself up and over it until you end up in a push-up position, with your shins resting on the ball. Your hands should be shoulder-width apart and legs about hip-width apart.

2 Engage your core and pull your knees into your chest as far as you can by contracting your abs, rolling the ball underneath your legs. Hold, then return to the starting position to repeat for the desired number of reps.

SWISS BALL PLANK

(with 'stirring the pot')

SETS	REPS	REST
3	20–30 seconds	30–45 seconds

1 Get into a plank position with your elbows resting on a Swiss ball and your chest resting on your forearms. Stabilise yourself with your feet either hip- or shoulder-width apart. Once balanced, lift your chest up and away from the ball, so your body weight is now supported by your forearms only (your legs are just for balance here). Contract your abs and squeeze your glutes. Don't allow your lower back to arch.

2 Start to roll the ball with your arms in small circles, both clockwise and anti-clockwise, challenging your core to stabilise you. If this is too difficult, just hold the plank position for the desired time.

AIRDYNE BIKE

SETS	REPS	REST
5	60 seconds	60 seconds

1 Set yourself up on an Airdyne bike and begin to cycle gently for 60 seconds, working at roughly 50% of your maximum effort.

2 Once you hit the 60-second mark, increase your intensity to roughly 90% for a further 60 seconds.

3 After that, drop the intensity back down to 50%. This is your active recovery period before you repeat the process a further 4 times. You're working to a '1 minute on, 1 minute off' protocol. (If your gym doesn't have an Airdyne bike, you can use a normal bike or an elliptical trainer.)

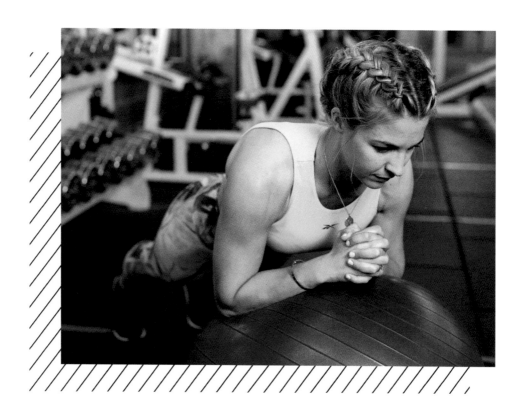

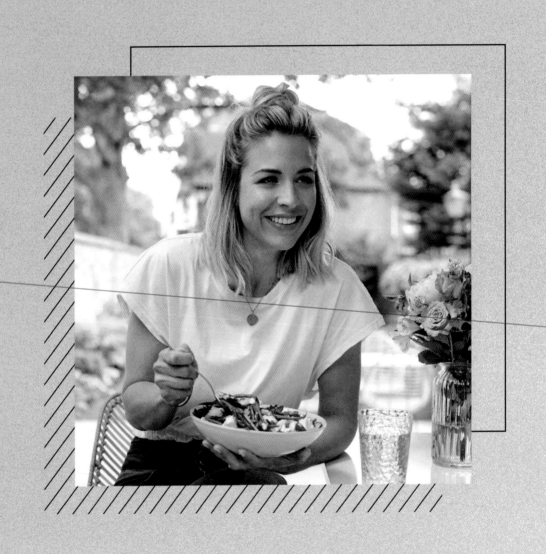

RECIPES

YOU ARE WHAT YOU EAT

Bored of feeling exhausted, run-down, bloated, hungry or – more likely – hangry?

Welcome to the life of any new mum. A healthy diet is often the first thing to go flying out the window upon the arrival of a baby. When you're busy propping your eyelids open with matchsticks, whipping up a 'square meal' can seem like an effort too far, especially with Deliveroo on speed dial. It's a catch-22 situation, though: when you eat crap, you feel like crap – and, over time, also begin to look like crap. You know the saying, 'You are what you eat'? Well, annoyingly, it's true!

I know when I used to feel awful, it was a lot harder to break the vicious cycle of eating rubbish. I'd find myself reaching for a sugary snack on autopilot, then suffering the blood sugar crash a couple of hours later, and needing more sugar or caffeine to climb back up again. The good news is, it is totally possible to break that cycle. You just need the right mindset – which you'll find by following this plan.

Eating well can change your life. By fuelling your body with delicious and nutritious food, you'll feel naturally more energetic and motivated, which will have a knock-on positive effect on your mood. You'll have the mental strength to play 9,000 games of 'roll the ball' without losing your mind, and you'll feel more determined to keep making good choices – like choosing to continue with your new training plan (see page 52).

In this section, you'll find breakfasts, snacks, light meals and lunches, dinners, desserts and drinks, all designed to speedily and easily give you the maximum nutritional content – to provide the right stuff in the right amount of time. And the best thing is, they taste delicious! Healthy food doesn't have to be bland and boring.

Who are these recipes for?

These recipes are suitable for all adults and children over the age of one, once they have been weaned. You'll find a mix of meat-based, vegetarian and vegan options, as well as veggie and vegan substitute ingredients where possible. I'm a vegetarian myself: I stopped eating red meat around ten years ago, and then gave up fish and chicken in the summer of 2019. I've been a fully-fledged veggie ever since and haven't looked back. That's what feels right for me, for my body and for my beliefs. However, I feel strongly that everyone's dietary decisions are entirely their own, and so this book should appease every foodie! Gorka eats meat and Mia enjoys a mixture of everything – I have no issues with cooking meat for her, and she loves my vegan and veggie dishes, too. She can make up her own mind when she's older.

If you're cooking for a family with very young kids, here are some nutritional guidelines to bear in mind:

- **Always adjust the portion size.**

- **Don't add extra salt during cooking.**

- **Kids under the age of one shouldn't have honey.**

- **Puddings shouldn't be encouraged. Go for fruit and/or yoghurt instead.**

Kids under the age of two need the concentrated energy and vitamins provided by fat. Therefore, energy-dense foods like whole milk, yoghurt and cheese are important. Once your child is two, you can gradually introduce lower-fat dairy products, but until then, their Tasmanian devil-style energy requirements need the full-fat versions. And while it's OK to have wholegrain foods (e.g. brown rice) occasionally, young kids should generally eat white starchy carbs to ensure they don't get full before they've taken in all the calories and nutrients they need. It's important to note that this book isn't for kids or about kids – it's about you – so I won't go into more detail here on the hows, whats and whys of children's diets. However, if you do want more info, www.nhs.uk/live-well is the go-to site for solid nutritional advice.

What you'll be eating

You'll be munching tasty, healthy and filling food that will enable you to look after yourself and your family without thinking too much about it. As speed is of the essence, you'll find recipes that use frozen veg, frozen seafood and microwaveable rice. You'll also be able to use up all the leftover stuff lurking in the fridge and make things in bulk to freeze or use in multiple dishes (such as my Ratatouille on page 242: great on its own, arguably even better as a jacket potato topping or stir-through pasta sauce).

The recipes aren't about being fancy or impressing the neighbours – although many will, which is always satisfying – they're about igniting a love for cooking by learning it's possible to make nutritious meals under pressure. You'll learn tips and tricks that will change your shopping habits forever. For example, frozen spinach and frozen blueberries are absolute game-changers – and can both be used to make kickass smoothies. No, I haven't lost my mind. Check it out on pages 266 and 274.

How to choose your meals

The recipes in my first book were based on a fat-loss goal. The entire idea was to lose fat and get lean in a realistic and manageable way. I therefore went into details on how to calculate your BMR (basal metabolic rate) and your TDEE (total daily energy expenditure) so you could work out the number of calories you'd need to consume per day in order to lose fat. Well, things have changed.

I know, and you know, that super-specific calorie counting is simply not feasible when you have a baby on one hip, a coffee in one hand and are about to trip over a plastic tractor. It's really not what you need to be thinking about right now. This book is not about fat loss – it's about feeling healthier, more energetic and more *you*. You may lose fat, but that'll be just one of the many benefits of a healthier lifestyle rather than the main goal.

NHS guidelines say that adult women require around 2,000 calories a day. You can use that as a framework when choosing dishes. (All the recipes list calorie calculation per portion. Please note, though, that where dishes have the option of different serving sizes (e.g. if the recipe serves 4–6), the calorie calculation has been based on the lower figure.) However, I'd much prefer you to focus on their nutritional value and make sure you're getting a balanced diet. That's why I've included detailed descriptions of food groups and nutrients here. Knowing this stuff is essential to understanding why certain meals make you feel either satisfied and energetic or bloated and sluggish. This is the info that will enable you to make educated, healthy choices.

CALORIE CALCULATION WHEN BREASTFEEDING

If you're exclusively breastfeeding, you'll require an extra 330 calories per day during the first six months of lactation. This should be reflected in a diet made up of nutrient-dense foods, as nutritional requirements are high during this time. However, whether you're breastfeeding or not, it's still important to eat a varied and balanced diet.

Another way of eating healthily

I'm a strong believer in eating mindfully: really focusing on what you're eating and how you're eating it. All too often, we just wolf down whatever's in front of us, barely registering it, let alone tasting it. Not only can this be bad for digestion, but also it can lead to us not making good food decisions because we're eating on autopilot. While you're following this plan, please try to:

- **pause between bites**

- **take smaller mouthfuls**

- **chew thoroughly**

- **ask yourself: 'What flavours am I tasting? What's the texture of the food like?'**

- **avoid distractions (ha ha!)**

'Oh sure!' you're thinking. 'It's easy to avoid distractions with a newborn strapped to my belly and a toddler swinging on the lampshade...' And that would be entirely fair. However, I mean avoid *unnecessary* distractions: try not to eat in front of the TV; try to make mealtimes screen-free; try not to eat while working. Rather than eating on the go or at the same time as doing something else, try to make it an 'event'. Say to yourself: 'This is officially lunchtime/dinnertime.' Also, listen to your body! Are you actually hungry, or are you only eating because you're bored, stressed or anxious? Being mindful means being present and aware of your choices. I want you to enjoy your food, and that means actually paying attention to what you're eating and why.

Ensuring your diet is balanced

The reason polishing off meatballs morning, noon and night isn't a solid plan is because different foods provide the different vitamins, minerals and nutrients that your body needs. That's why it's really important to mix things up and try to incorporate as many different foods from each food group as possible when choosing what to eat. Each main meal should ideally be based around these five food groups: carbohydrates, proteins, fats (including oils and spreads), fruit and veg, and dairy. Obviously that's not always possible or realistic, so I've provided tips within many of the recipe introductions for ways to sneak in extra nutrients or balance things out with snacks.

THE FIVE GROUPS

1 / CARBOHYDRATES

Forget any chat you've heard that all carbs are bad. Carbohydrates are macronutrients and are essential to your diet. There are three main types found in food: starch, fibre and sugar. Here, we'll go through all three.

- **STARCHY CARBS**

  Starchy carbs are an important source of energy. When digested, they break down into glucose: the body's main energy fuel source. Glucose is essential to keep the brain functioning. Examples of starchy carbs include potatoes, pasta, rice, bread, couscous, oats and grains, like rye, millet and buckwheat. They often have a bad reputation for being fattening, but that's typically linked to what they're served with or how they're cooked, e.g. cheesy pasta, pizza, buttery potatoes or deep-fried chips. Starchy carbs should make up around a third of the food on your plate, which is why a lot of classic meals have them as a 'base' – think mashed potato on a fish pie, pasta in lasagne or rice to accompany a curry. You should aim to eat three to four servings of starchy carbohydrates per day.

- **FIBRE**

  Fibre is the catch-all name for carbs found in plant-based foods – like fruit and veg, nuts, seeds, peas, beans, cereals and pulses – that aren't digested or absorbed by the body but pass straight through, helping to keep your digestive system healthy and prevent constipation. Eating plenty of higher-fibre foods is associated with a lower risk of heart disease and bowel cancer.

  Wholegrain varieties of carbs are higher in fibre, which is why I mostly use wholemeal pasta, bread or rice. Potatoes with their skins are a good source of fibre, too. A small handful of dried fruit, nuts and seeds (up to 30g) or some veg crudités are great fibre-rich snacking options. Those aged seventeen and over should aim for 30g fibre per day, to keep things, um, flowing nicely (gross). If you follow a healthy, varied diet, that shouldn't be a problem.

- **SUGAR**

  There are two main types of sugars: added sugar and natural sugar.

  Added sugar is – surprise, surprise – sugar that is added to food and drinks by the manufacturer. It's often found in foods that provide little in the way of other nutrients, e.g. fizzy drinks and sweets. Natural sugar is similarly self-explanatory: it's sugar that occurs – yep, you guessed it – naturally in foods like fruit, some veg and even milk and yoghurt. It's added sugar you want to reduce in your diet, as it can increase the risk of tooth decay and contribute to health problems. It can be difficult to differentiate between sugars on many food labels, as often manufacturers clump added and natural sugars together under a category called 'of which sugars', which is frustrating. That's why, ideally, it's always better to use fresh and natural ingredients – like we do in this book! – so you know exactly what you're eating.

2/ PROTEIN

Protein is an incredibly hard-working macronutrient that plays an essential role in forming and maintaining bones, muscles, cartilage, skin, nails, hair and blood. It also builds and repairs tissues and enzymes, and aids the function of hormones and other chemicals. You could say it's the star player of nutrients, but actually, it only reaches its full potential when consumed as part of a balanced diet – it needs the rest of the team to win. (Sorry for the laboured sports reference there – but hey, I enjoyed it.)

The science bit: proteins are large molecules made up of long chains of amino acids. Our bodies only produce what are known as 'non-essential amino acids' (NEAA), so we must get the others – the essential ones (EAA) from food.

The main protein sources are red meat, fish, eggs, beans, lentils, poultry, nuts, seeds and meat alternatives, such as tofu. How much protein women need depends on many factors. Typically, 0.8–1.2g of protein per kilogram of body weight per day would be a good maintenance intake. However, for those looking to maintain muscle mass while training – and potentially to increase it – it's wise to consume between 1.2–1.6g protein per kilogram of body weight per day. Try to choose leaner proteins – and note that they tend to work best when they come from different sources. For example, eating a combination of plant proteins can boost and complement their biological

effectiveness within the body.

3/ FATS

The main types of fat found in food are saturated and unsaturated fat. Saturated fats are commonly thought of as 'bad' fats and can be found in foods like butter, cream and cakes. Eating too much of this type of fat can lead to increased cholesterol (a risk factor for heart disease). Meanwhile, unsaturated – or 'good' fat – can be found in things like vegetable oils (e.g. rapeseed or sunflower oil), oily fish (e.g. salmon and mackerel), eggs, avocados and some nuts. Aim to eat less saturated fat and more unsaturated, as the latter is essential for helping the body to absorb vitamins A, D, E and K. It also helps to regulate hormones, provide energy, reduce cell inflammation, protect organs, maintain cell membranes and keep the brain ticking along.

- **OMEGA-3 FATTY ACIDS**
  Fish is a protein food, but it also contains omega-3 fatty acids, which are essential for health. The body can't produce omega-3 on its own, so has to get it from food or supplements. In the UK, adults are advised to eat two portions of fish each week, with at least one portion being an oily fish like trout, mackerel or salmon. Vegetarians and vegans can find omega-3 in chia seeds, ground flaxseed, flaxseed oil and nuts (especially walnuts). Pregnant and breastfeeding women should eat no more than two portions of oily fish per week. While the omega-3 helps develop a baby's brain, eyes and nerves, oily fish contains low-level pollutants that may build up in the body and affect the future development of the baby.

4/ FRUIT AND VEGETABLES

If you thought the phrase 'eat the rainbow' was about Skittles, I'm sorry to disappoint you. It's actually about fruit and veg! Eating different coloured fruit and vegetables provides you with different vitamins and minerals. 'Eating the rainbow', therefore, means mixing up your diet, for example by eating green broccoli and red apples, purple beetroot and orange peppers. Fruit and vegetables are best eaten in season, when at their most ripe, juicy and sweet.

The World Health Organization (WHO) recommends getting a minimum of 'five a day' (five portions of fruit and vegetables, which equates to roughly 400g) to lower the risk of serious health problems. It may sound like a lot, but remember: all fruit and vegetables count, whether they're fresh, tinned, dried or frozen. The one exception is white potatoes, which are a starchy carb. I'd recommend aiming for a minimum of two fruit and three veg portions per day.

5/ DAIRY

Cheese, plain milk and yoghurt are important sources of nutrients including calcium, protein and iodine. You can make healthier choices, where possible, by opting for plain or lower-fat versions, always checking the label to ensure they're not high in added sugar. For vegans, or those with a cow's milk allergy or a lactose intolerance, unsweetened, calcium-fortified dairy alternatives, such as plant-based milk and yoghurt, are good replacements. I'm a big fan of unsweetened almond milk and coconut milk. You can also get great vegan cheese options nowadays. Aim for two to three servings of dairy per day, for example 200ml semi-skimmed milk or 4 tablespoons of natural yoghurt.

TAKEN WITH A PINCH OF SALT

How much salt is too much salt – and should we care? Sodium, a mineral found in salt (aka sodium chloride), is needed for nerve and muscle function, and helps regulate the amount of fluid in our cells. However, in large quantities, salt can raise blood pressure, which, in turn, can increase the risk of cardiovascular disease (e.g. heart attacks and strokes). Foods that are naturally high in salt include bacon, olives, cheese, ham, gravy and stock. Salt is also added to many common staple foods, like bread and breakfast cereal. (This isn't to say you can't eat these types of foods – just be mindful of their salt content and check the food label.)

Salt was originally added to food for preservation purposes, but ever since the invention of fridges, we haven't needed it for that. However, we still sprinkle it liberally on our food. In the UK, adults should have no more than 6g salt per day (less for children) and it's very easy to exceed these requirements if you're adding it to food unnecessarily. Fresh and dried herbs and spices, as well as ingredients such as garlic, chilli, ginger and lemon, are great alternative culinary weapons for boosting flavour.

Drink to your own health

CAFFEINE

There is no official recommended daily caffeine intake for adults, but it can affect us all differently, so tune into how your own body – and mood – respond on days your intake is high, and adjust things accordingly. Don't forget there is also caffeine in tea (including green tea), soft drinks, energy drinks and chocolate. Decaffeinated tea and coffee or herbal drinks are great alternatives.

For breastfeeding women, evidence shows that caffeine consumption should be limited to a maximum of 200mg per day (the same applies during pregnancy). This is the equivalent of two mugs of instant coffee.

ALCOHOL

On this plan, I'm going to ask that you don't drink alcohol for twelve weeks. Before you call the fun police, hear me out. Alcohol is empty calories, providing minimal nutritional value. It slows down the recovery and repair process after exercise by inhibiting the function of hormones that aid that process, and it's also a diuretic, contributing to dehydration. Booze is usually drunk during social occasions when you'll be feeling less motivated to stick to your healthy goals, especially if you're surrounded by salty and sugary snacks. And, on top of all of that, it's a depressant, meaning it can lead to you feeling low and anxious. It also impairs cognitive function, making you feel slow and sluggish. It's basically the antithesis of everything we're promoting in this book. Sure, one beer on a sunny afternoon isn't going to upend your progress, but you've done nine months booze-free before now, so what's another twelve weeks in order to see, feel and enjoy real change?

On this plan, I'm going to ask that you don't drink alcohol for twelve weeks. Before you call the fun police, hear me out...

Vitamins and minerals

The information here refers to advice given to parents and children over the age of one. For more info on vitamin recommendations for babies (and just in general), please visit www.nhs.uk/conditions/vitamins-and-minerals.

VITAMIN D

Vitamin D can be found in egg yolks, oily fish and fortified foods such as breakfast cereals – however, it's impossible to get enough of it from food alone. The main source, of course, is the sun! Usually, we'd all get enough of the good stuff from April to September to see us through the winter, but in 2020, after lockdown scuppered everyone's plans for spending time outside, public health advice regarding vitamin D changed. At the time of writing, it's therefore advised that, while all kids under four should still take vitamin D supplements (as was always the case), adults and children over the age of four should also now consider taking a 10mcg supplement every day for the foreseeable future (previously this was just for October to March). However, this recommendation may have changed again by the time you read this (these are strange times we live in!), so please check for the most up-to-date information.

IODINE

According to the European Food Safety Authority, adults need 150mcg iodine per day, while breastfeeding or pregnant women require 200mcg per day. Vegetarians or vegans may be at greater risk of a deficiency as the most iodine-rich foods are fish, shellfish, eggs and dairy products. However, they should be able to find it in certain fortified, plant-based dairy alternatives, such as oat milk and oat yoghurt (Oatly, for example, fortifies many of its products with iodine).

CALCIUM

Calcium is integral for maintaining bone density. Adult women require 700mg calcium per day, but an additional 550mg per day is needed when breastfeeding. (30g Cheddar, 200ml cow's milk and a single medium-sized orange equate to approximately 550mg calcium.)

PLANT MILKS

I've used a lot of fortified and unsweetened plant milks (e.g. almond, oat and cashew) in these recipes, because they contain lots of vitamins and minerals. (Rice milk is another option, although it's not suitable for kids under five.) Check the labels, keeping a keen eye out for those fortified with vitamin D, iodine, iron, calcium and B vitamins such as vitamins B2 (riboflavin) and B12.

VITAMIN B12

Vitamin B12 is typically found in meat, fish, eggs, dairy products and specially fortified foods. For vegans, other sources include breakfast cereals, unsweetened plant-milk drinks and fortified yeast extract. If you're a vegan and concerned about a deficiency, speak with your doctor.

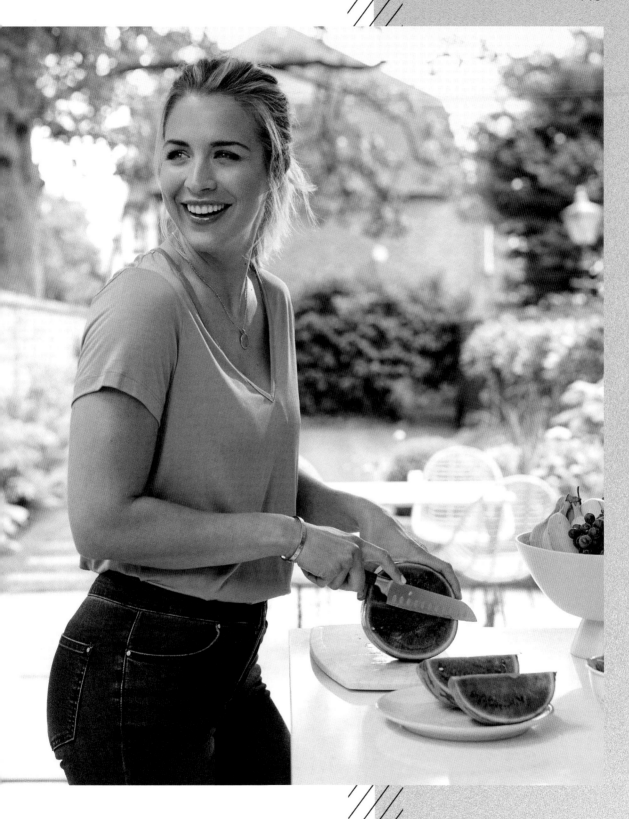

The Ultimate Body Plan for New Mums

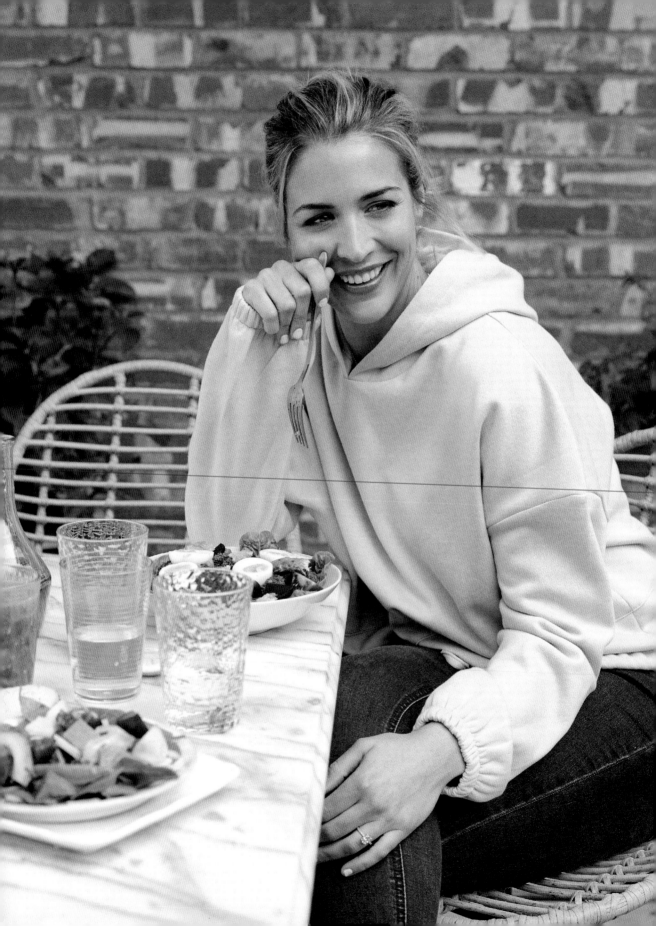

Tracking

On page 75, you'll find your Progress Table. I'd like you to copy this out in a notebook and fill it in every day. There, you can keep track of how you feel, both mentally and physically, at the start and end of each day, and you can also track your meals and workouts. This table is an integral part of the programme, enabling you to spot patterns connecting your mood, behaviour and body. For example, on days you feel low or anxious in the morning, are you more likely to skip training and eat badly? If so, how does that affect how you feel at the end of the day? If, instead of skipping training, you still do it, does that have a positive knock-on effect on your mood and food choices? You'll be able to see how you respond emotionally to different events, and how that affects your choices when it comes to exercising and eating. It's all connected. This awareness will enable you to interrupt negative patterns and change them for more positive ones. And, by noting down your meals, you'll be able to work out if any particular ingredients agree or disagree with you. It will also help you make sure you're mixing things up and getting a balanced diet.

Above all though, filling in this table is about making a commitment to yourself to take the plan seriously. You are less likely to skip training or eat crap if you know you have to write it down. That's a fact. And the best bit is, you'll be able to look back at your table throughout the twelve weeks and see the progress you're making in black and white. What a huge achievement that will be. (And remember to reward yourself for it, too! See page 51.)

You are less likely to skip training or eat crap if you know you have to write it down. That's a fact.

BREAKFASTS

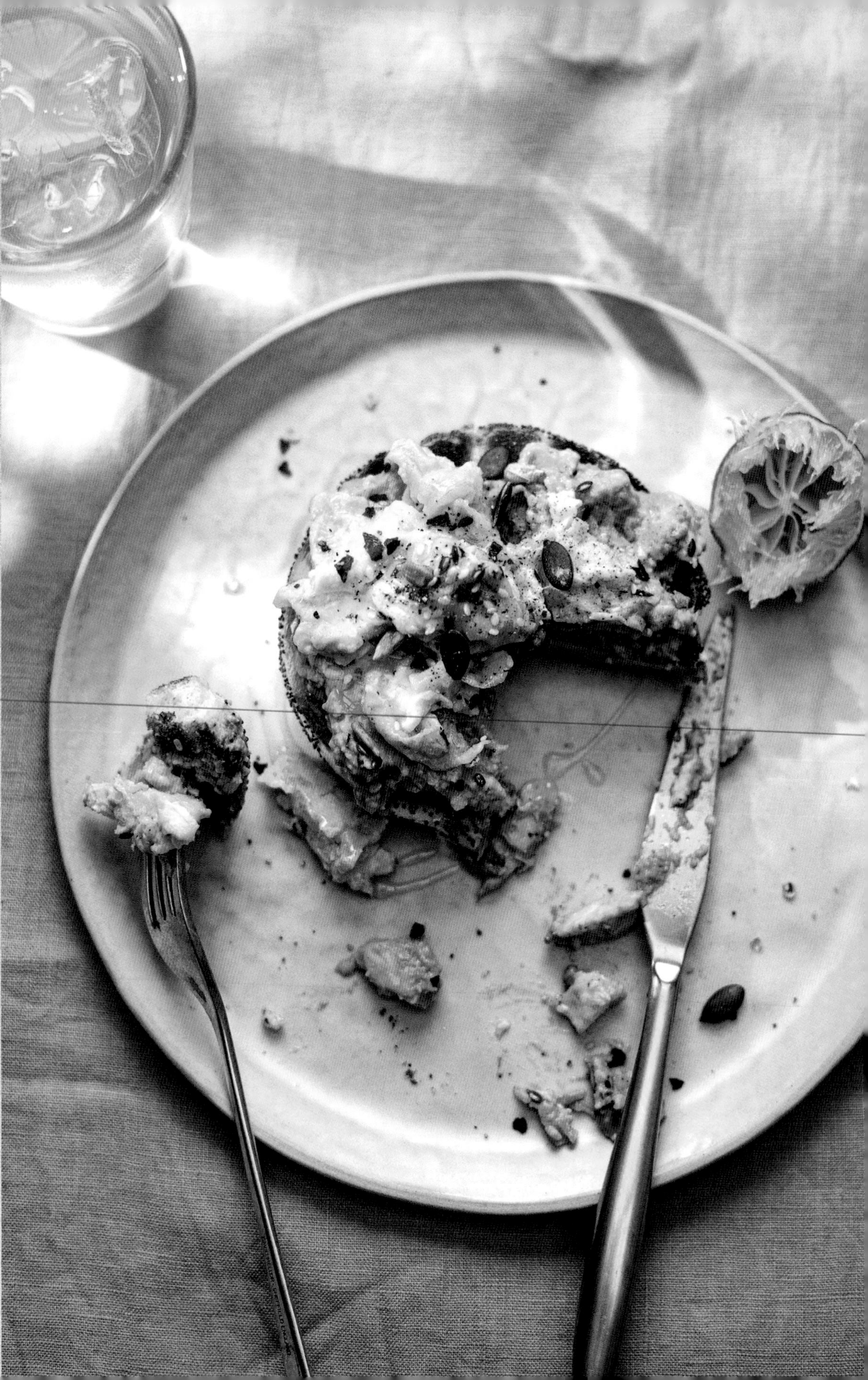

toasted bagels with scrambled eggs, chilli avocado & seeds

Prep time:
2 minutes

Cooking time:
3 minutes

Calories per serving:
387

I always go for wholemeal or seeded bagels as they contain about twice as much fibre per 100g as the plain white ones. For this recipe, make sure the avocados are ripe, otherwise they're tough to mash and actually taste pretty horrible. I also always keep a jar of mixed seeds handy to sprinkle on top. They add a nice bit of extra protein – and add a crunch that contrasts well with the soft egg and avocado.

serves 2

1 avocado, peeled, stoned and cut into chunks

pinch of chilli flakes, plus extra to serve (optional)

juice of 1 lime

sea salt and freshly ground black pepper

1 wholemeal bagel, halved

1 tablespoon olive oil

2 large free-range eggs, whisked

1 tablespoon mixed seeds (I love a mix of pumpkin, sunflower and chia seeds)

1/ Place the avocado chunks in a bowl and mash with a fork. Stir in the chilli flakes and lime juice. Taste and season as needed.

2/ Toast the bagel. While it's toasting, heat the oil in a medium-sized frying pan over a medium heat. Add the eggs and cook for 2 minutes, stirring occasionally, until the scrambled eggs are cooked through but still slightly wobbly.

3/ Top each half of the toasted bagel with mashed chilli and lime avocado. Divide the scrambled eggs between the bagel halves and finish with a sprinkling of mixed seeds (and an extra pinch of chilli flakes, if you fancy!)

blueberry & peanut protein porridge

Prep time:
2 minutes

Cooking time:
5–6 minutes

Calories per serving:
282

This blueberry protein porridge satisfies hunger and keeps energy levels up for ages. Sprinkle nuts and chia seeds on top for some added protein oomph to keep you going. (This should be eaten two hours before training, FYI.) Here's a handy tip: blueberries keep well in the freezer and can be popped straight into porridges and smoothies.

serves 4

85g rolled oats

240ml water

240ml unsweetened fortified almond or cashew milk

150g frozen blueberries

3 tablespoons good-quality peanut/other nut butter

30g almonds, roughly chopped

1 teaspoon chia seeds (optional)

a drizzle of runny honey, to sweeten (optional)

1/ Place a medium-sized non-stick saucepan over a medium heat. Add the oats, water, milk and 100g of the frozen blueberries. Cook for 5–6 minutes, stirring occasionally, then stir through 2 tablespoons of the peanut butter.

2/ Divide the porridge between 4 bowls and top each serving with the almonds and chia seeds (if using), and the remaining blueberries and peanut butter.

3/ Drizzle over a little honey if you like it a bit sweeter.

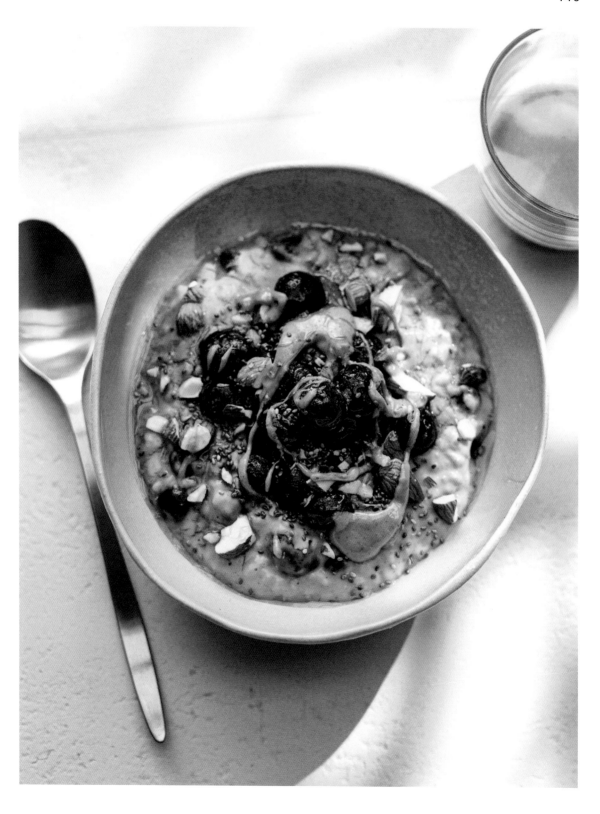

The Ultimate Body Plan for New Mums

cinnamon & fig overnight oats

Prep time:
5 minutes, plus
overnight chilling

Calories per serving:
360

This recipe is great to prep the night before when you know you have a busy morning ahead. It's also ideal for kids who are weaning – as long as the nuts are ground or crushed (to avoid a choking hazard). Consider stirring in some grated apple or peanut butter, and throwing some berries on top.

serves 4

100g rolled oats

250ml unsweetened fortified almond milk, plus extra if needed

4 figs, chopped into chunks

2 tablespoons nuts of your choice, crushed or ground

pinch of ground cinnamon

1/ Place the oats in a plastic container and cover with the almond milk. Add half the figs. Cover and leave overnight in the fridge.

2/ In the morning, give the oats a good stir to mix it all up, adding an extra splash of milk if you want it loose

3/ Top with the nuts and remaining figs, sprinkle with cinnamon and enjoy.

chocolate & banana porridge

Prep time:
2 minutes

Cooking time:
5–6 minutes

Calories per serving:
354

Instead of 'real' chocolate, this recipe uses cocoa powder. It contains absolutely no sugar whatsoever, yet still provides that gorgeous smooth flavour. Starting the day with a banana will not only deliver an energy boost – they're an excellent source of carbs, potassium and vitamin B6 – it will also tick off one of your five a day. (This is also a neat way of tricking kids into thinking they're getting chocolate for breakfast...)

serves 2

85g rolled oats

200ml unsweetened fortified oat milk

2 bananas, 1 mashed and 1 sliced

1 tablespoon cocoa powder

good pinch of cinnamon, plus extra to serve

1 tablespoon runny honey

1/ Place a non-stick saucepan over a medium heat and add the oats, milk, mashed banana, cocoa powder and cinnamon.

2/ Stir to combine and cook for 5–6 minutes, stirring occasionally so it doesn't stick to the pan. If the mixture is too thick or needs loosening, add a splash of water.

3/ Serve the porridge in 2 bowls, and top each one with banana slices, a drizzle of honey and a pinch of cinnamon.

turmeric tofu scramble with mango yoghurt

Prep time:
5 minutes

Cooking time:
15–20 minutes

Calories per serving:
393

Turmeric is an amazing spice that, in my humble opinion, is not used enough. Commonly found in curries, it adds a subtle, earthy flavour to the dish, as well as a brilliant yellow colour. This is a proper show-off breakfast, so I recommend presenting it to overnight guests in the morning and acting all modest when they tell you how impressed they are.

serves 4

1 tablespoon olive oil, plus extra if needed

1 small red onion, cut into wedges

1 large potato, cut into 2cm cubes

225g smoked firm tofu

¼ teaspoon ground turmeric

50g fresh spinach

sea salt and freshly ground black pepper

4 tablespoons natural yoghurt

1 tablespoon mango chutney

4 small wholemeal wraps

1/ Heat the oil in a frying pan over a medium heat. Add the onion and potato and cook for 5 minutes until everything is getting nice and golden. Add a good splash of water and cover with a lid, then cook for a further 5 minutes.

2/ Move the onion and potato over to one side of the pan, then crumble the tofu into the other side. Add the turmeric to the tofu and stir through. Once the tofu is coated, stir everything in the pan together carefully for a further 5 minutes (you might need to add a little extra oil).

3/ Add the spinach to the pan and toss everything together until the spinach has wilted. Season to taste.

4/ In a bowl, mix together the yoghurt and mango chutney. Lightly toast the wraps (or warm through in a frying pan over a medium heat).

5/ Divide the tofu scramble between 4 plates and serve, with a dollop of the yoghurt chutney and toasted wraps on the side, for dunking.

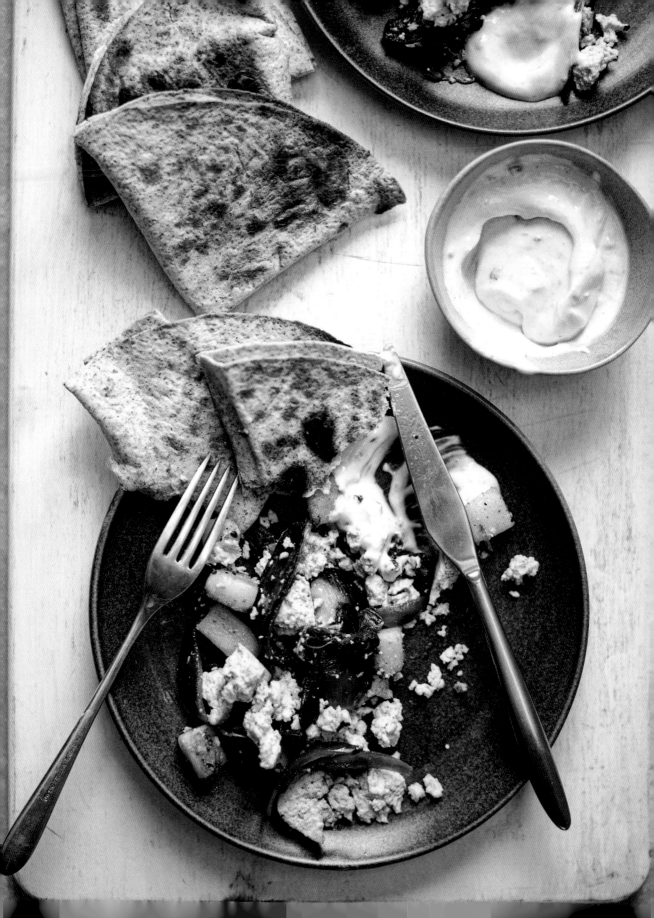

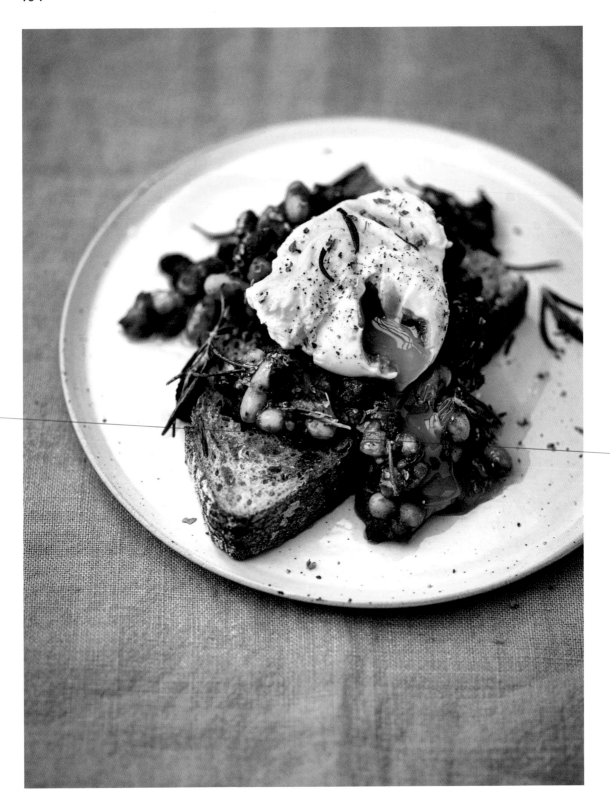

posh beans on toast

Baked beans get a makeover. Sure, this takes a little more effort than cracking a tin open, but it's totally worth it for the flavour. This recipe makes a big batch, so you can reheat it later in a pan, just as you would 'normal' beans. I've used black beans and cannellini beans here, but butter beans or chickpeas will work just as well.

Prep time:
5 minutes

Cooking time:
13 minutes

Calories per serving:
316

serves 4

1 tablespoon olive oil, plus extra for drizzling (optional)

2 garlic cloves, sliced

pinch of dried rosemary or oregano (or 1 sprig, finely chopped)

1 teaspoon smoked paprika

1 x 400g tin cannellini beans, drained

1 x 400g tin black beans, drained

1 x 400g tin chopped tomatoes

sea salt and freshly ground black pepper

4 free-range eggs

4 slices of wholemeal bread

a few rosemary sprigs (optional)

1/ Heat the oil in a medium-sized non-stick saucepan over a medium heat. Add the garlic, rosemary and smoked paprika and cook for 3 minutes, stirring continuously.

2/ Add the cannellini beans, black beans and tinned tomatoes, and carry on cooking for 10 minutes, stirring occasionally, until thick. Season with salt and pepper.

3/ Meanwhile, cook the eggs to your liking and toast the bread.

4/ Pile the beans onto the toast and top with the eggs. If you're feeling extra fancy, drizzle over a little olive oil and sprinkle with some rosemary before serving.

avocado & spinach smoothie bowl

Prep time:
5 minutes

Calories per serving:
314

Having a smoothie in a bowl feels much more fun (and substantial) than in a boring glass. Top with whatever you like, but I recommend balancing the savoury taste with sweeter fruits. If your blender's seen better days, either choose the smaller cauliflower florets or (after running them under the tap to defrost slightly) roughly chop them up beforehand, as they're notoriously tricky to blend.

serves 2

120g frozen cauliflower florets

handful of spinach (about 30g)

½ ripe avocado, peeled and stoned

150ml unsweetened fortified almond, oat or other dairy-free milk, plus extra if needed

1 tablespoon runny honey

2 kiwi fruits, peeled and chopped

2 dates, stoned and torn

50g blueberries

1 tablespoon nut butter

1 teaspoon mixed seeds

1/ Place the cauliflower, spinach, avocado, milk and honey in a high-powered blender. Blend until smooth, adding a splash more milk if the mixture is too thick.

2/ Pour the smoothie into bowls, then top with the kiwi fruits, dates, blueberries, nut butter and seeds. Tuck in.

baked apples & pears with yoghurt

Prep time:
5 minutes

Cooking time:
50 minutes

Calories per serving:
256

This tastes great whether eaten immediately or saved for the next day (when it can be enjoyed warm or cold). Simply prep the fruit, shove it in the oven and then forget about it for a while. I always serve with a dollop of yoghurt – you can even mix things up by blitzing the fruit after cooking to make a purée.

serves 4

500g ripe pears (Conference pears work well), peeled, cored and cut into wedges

500g eating apples (Braeburn or Cox are my favourites), peeled, cored and cut into wedges

150ml apple juice

1 cinnamon stick

500g Greek yoghurt

1/ Preheat the oven to 200°C/180°C fan/400°F/gas 6.

2/ Place the pears and apples in a roasting tray. Pour over the apple juice and add the cinnamon stick.

3/ Cover with tin foil and cook for 40 minutes or until the fruit is softened and smelling delicious. Remove the foil and cook for a further 10 minutes.

4/ Divide the yoghurt between 4 bowls and top each one with a serving of the baked fruit.

turkish eggs

Prep time:
5 minutes

Cooking time:
6 minutes

Calories per serving:
392

Another impressive-looking breakfast that takes hardly any time to prepare. You'll need some good-quality hummus (extra points go to those who use their own home-made version; see page 173), and make sure you don't overcook the eggs – they should come out silky, not hard. If you live near any Turkish shops, use some of their lovely breads. Otherwise, a wholemeal wrap will do.

serves 2

2 large free-range eggs

2 soft Turkish flatbreads or small wholemeal wraps

4 tablespoons Butter Bean Hummus (page 173) or shop-bought hummus

2 handfuls of spinach

pinch of smoked paprika, or sumac if you have it

extra-virgin olive oil, for drizzling

sea salt and freshly ground black pepper

1/ Fill a saucepan with water and place over a high heat. Bring to the boil, then add the eggs and boil for 6 minutes. Remove the eggs from the pan using a slotted spoon and run under cold water for a few minutes. Allow to cool a little, then carefully peel off the shells.

2/ Meanwhile, lightly toast the flatbreads (or warm through in a frying pan over a medium heat), then spread 2 tablespoons of hummus over each one and top with a handful of spinach.

3/ Quarter the peeled boiled eggs and place on top of the spinach. Sprinkle with smoked paprika or sumac, drizzle with extra-virgin olive oil and season to taste with a little salt and pepper before serving.

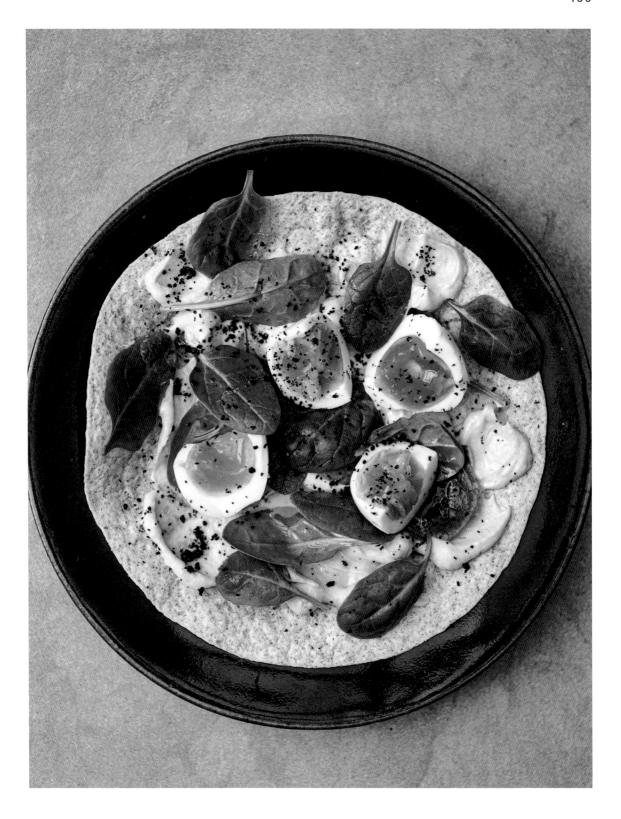

The Ultimate Body Plan for New Mums

portobello mushrooms on toast

Prep time:
2 minutes

Cooking time:
8 minutes

Calories per serving:
293

As strange as it sounds, portobello mushrooms are really meaty – they make for great meat substitutes in dishes like beef Wellington, for example. If you can't get hold of any, don't worry: chestnut or button mushrooms will also work here. Just be sure to slice them as thickly as possible. You should get four slices out of a chestnut mushroom, while buttons will be fine halved.

serves 2

1 tablespoon olive oil

350g portobello mushrooms, sliced

2 large free-range eggs (optional)

2 garlic cloves, finely sliced

50g spinach

sea salt and freshly ground black pepper

2 slices of wholemeal bread

butter, for spreading

1/ Heat the oil in a medium-sized non-stick frying pan over a medium heat. Add the mushrooms and cook for 5 minutes, stirring occasionally.

2/ Meanwhile, prepare the eggs (if using). Place a small saucepan of water over a high heat and bring to the boil, then reduce the heat to a low simmer. Use a spoon to carefully swirl the water around, then crack one of the eggs into the middle of the swirl. Crack the other egg into the water soon after, then poach the eggs for 3 minutes. Remove with a slotted spoon and set aside on a plate lined with kitchen paper to drain.

3/ Add the garlic and spinach to the pan with the mushrooms and season with salt and pepper. Stir until the spinach has wilted and the garlic is lightly golden.

4/ Meanwhile, toast and lightly butter the bread.

5/ To serve, pile the mushrooms onto the slices of toast and top each one with a poached egg, if using.

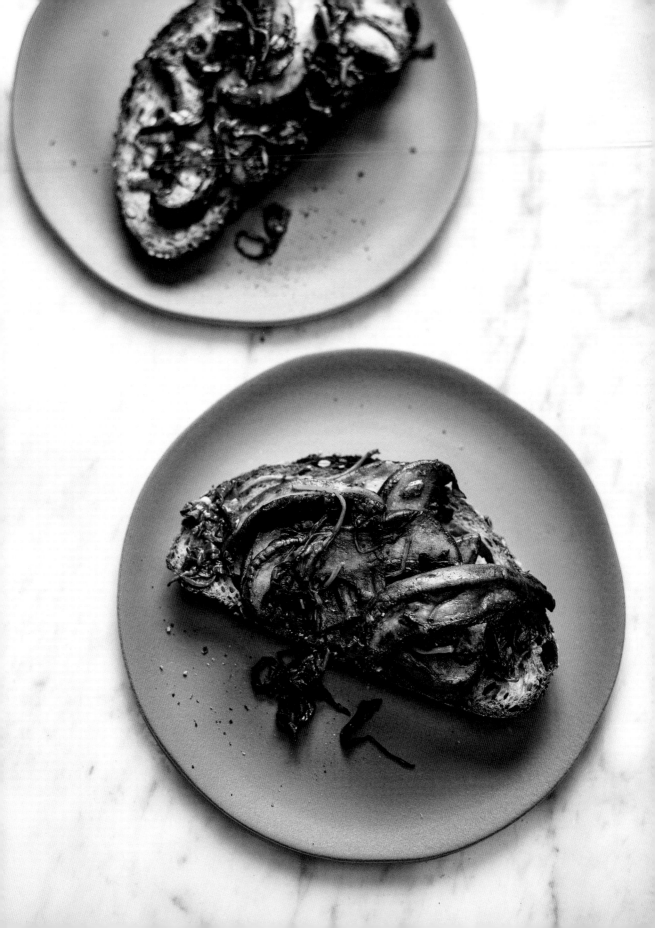

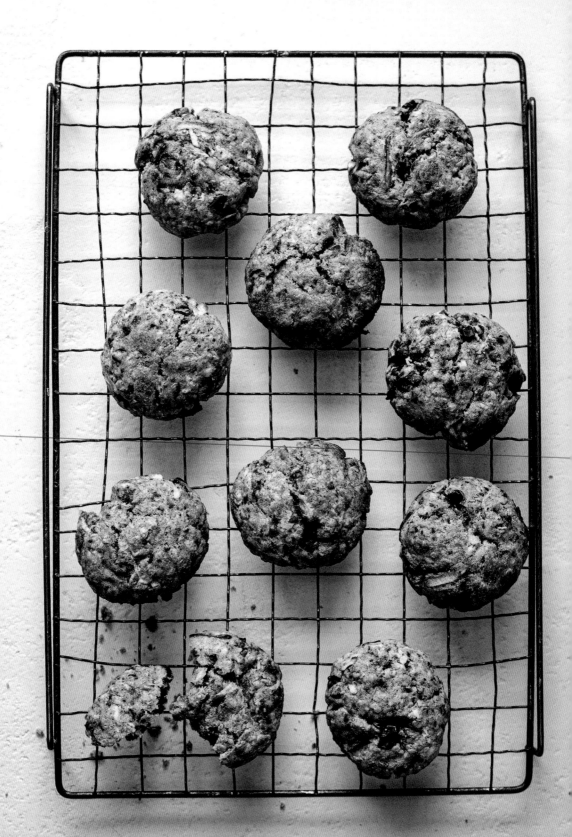

oaty apple & date cookies

Prep time:
8 minutes

Cooking time:
14–16 minutes

Calories per serving:
176

Older kids (older than your newborn, obvs) will love helping to make these delicious chewy cookies. If you don't have a food-processor, just use your hands to make rough breadcrumbs and then stir in the other ingredients to combine. You can use whatever dried fruit is hiding in your cupboards. If you swap in dairy-free butter and cacao nibs instead of chocolate, this recipe can be completely vegan.

makes 12 cookies

100g cold unsalted butter

125g wholemeal self-raising flour

100g dates, stoned

1 tablespoon maple syrup

50g dark chocolate (80% cocoa solids), cut into 1cm chunks

50g rolled oats

1 small apple, grated

1 teaspoon ground cinnamon (optional)

1 teaspoon chia seeds

approx. 1 tablespoon milk (semi-skimmed cow's milk, unsweetened fortified oat milk or whatever you fancy!)

1/ Preheat the oven to 200°C/180°C fan/400°F/gas 6 and line two baking trays with baking paper.

2/ Place the butter, flour, dates and maple syrup in a food-processor and pulse until the mixture forms rough breadcrumbs.

3/ Transfer the mixture to a bowl and add the chocolate, oats, grated apple, cinnamon (if using) and chia seeds. Mix together using a wooden spoon, then add a splash of the milk. The dough should come together into a ball – add a little more milk if it is not coming together.

4/ Take the dough and roll it into a thick sausage, then divide in half. Slice each half into 6 pieces, so you have 12 in total. Roll each piece of dough into a ball and check to make sure they are evenly sized.

5/ Place the dough balls on the prepared baking trays and gently push down so they form 5cm rounds. They will expand slightly as they bake, but not too much.

6/ Bake for 14–16 minutes, or until cooked through and golden all over. Leave the cookies to cool for 5 minutes on the baking trays, then carefully transfer to a cooling rack for a further 5 minutes before eating. These are delicious served on the same day with a cuppa. If keeping for a few days, store in an airtight container and see how long you can make the batch last!

mixed nut butter

Prep time:
15 minutes

Cooking time:
10 minutes

Calories per
tablespoon:
90

Yes, you can actually make your own nut butter! 'Why would I want to?' I hear you cry. Well, because the recipe is surprisingly simple, it works out cheaper than buying a pot of the stuff, you can make it in batches to keep (so it lasts longer) and you have total control over the ingredients. And, if all of that wasn't enough, it's also more environmentally friendly, as shop-bought nut butter normally comes in plastic pots.

This recipe is great for spreading on toast or bagels, or adding to smoothies for an additional protein kick. It's also perfect for dipping apples into. Yep. Simply core and slice an apple and dip it in – it's the snack that's been missing from your life.

makes 450g

450g mixed nuts (pecans, almonds and cashews all work really nicely)

1 tablespoon maple syrup or runny honey

pinch of sea salt

1/ Preheat the oven to 200°C/180°C fan/400°F/gas 6.

2/ Place the nuts on a large baking tray and roast for 10 minutes (checking halfway and giving them a shake), until toasted and smelling delicious.

3/ Remove from the oven and leave the nuts to cool for about 10 minutes, then transfer to the food-processor.

4/ Blend on full power for about 5 minutes until the mixture starts to become creamy. It will go all grainy first, then it will start forming clumps. Keep going – I promise it will become creamy!

5/ As you blend, add the maple syrup or honey and salt. Keep blending, scraping down the sides of the food-processor to make sure everything is combined.

6/ Let the mixture cool, as sometimes the blending generates some heat. Transfer the nut butter to a sterilised jar (see Tip) and keep in the fridge for up to 2 weeks.

TIP/ To sterilise a jar, simply wash it well with hot soapy water and rinse, then either place the jar in an oven preheated to 160°C/140°C fan/325°F/gas 3 for about 15 minutes, or submerge it in boiling water.

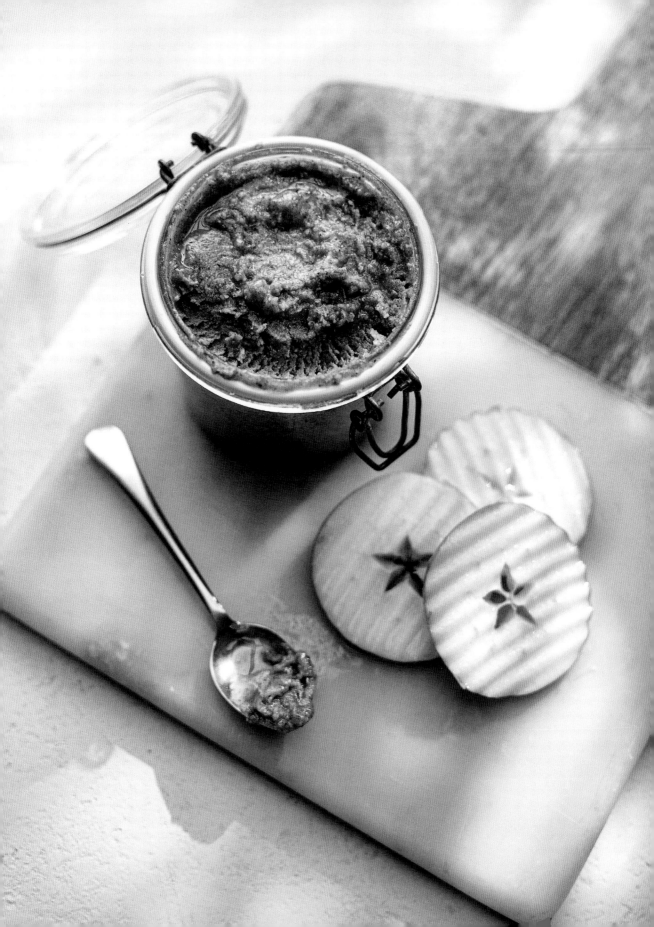

chocolate orange nutty bites

Prep time:
5 minutes (plus 30 minutes chilling)

Calories per ball:
112

The zesty orange and caramelly dates in this recipe deliver a satisfying, sticky flavour that is dangerously moreish. Medjool dates are ideal for this if you can get them. If you find the bites come out a little stodgy, the dates you've used may be too hard, so next time, add 1–2 tablespoons of water during step 3. I've found a jar of these bites make a lovely gift for new mums.

makes 20 balls

250g soft dates, stoned

100g almonds

1 tablespoon pumpkin seeds

2 tablespoons nut butter (shop-bought or home-made – see page 164)

1 tablespoon coconut oil

zest of 1 orange

pinch of sea salt

40g dark chocolate (80% cocoa solids), roughly chopped

1/ Line a baking tray with baking paper and set aside until needed.

2/ Put the dates, almonds and pumpkin seeds in a food-processor and blitz until well combined.

3/ Add the nut butter, coconut oil, orange zest and salt and blitz again to combine. If the mix feels too dry or isn't coming together, you can add 1–2 tablespoons cold water.

4/ Transfer the mixture to a bowl and add the chocolate chunks. Stir to combine, or just use your hands to scrunch it all together so it is evenly mixed through.

5/ Take tablespoons of the mixture and use your hands to roll them into balls – you should get about 20. Place on the prepared baking tray and chill in the fridge for 30 minutes.

6/ Once chilled, the balls are ready to eat – or you can transfer them to a large glass jar or container and keep in the fridge until you fancy one.

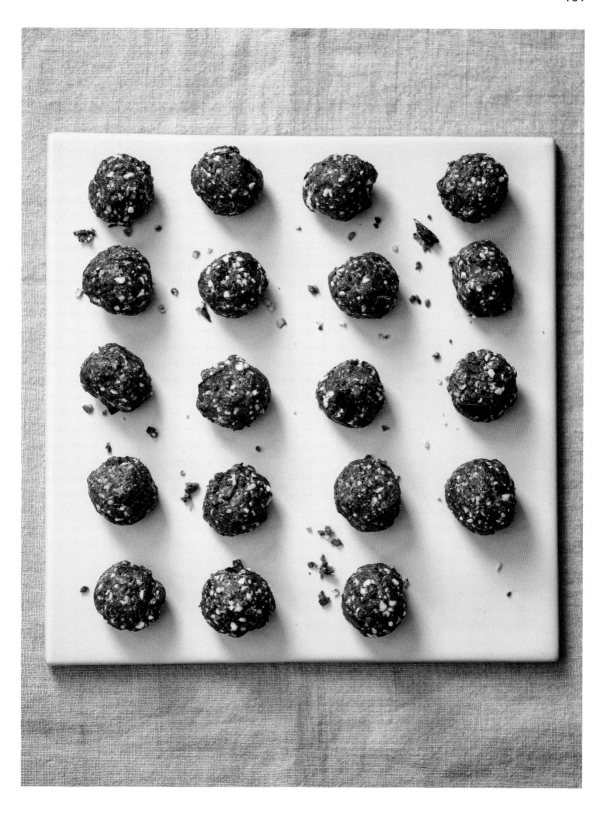

The Ultimate Body Plan for New Mums

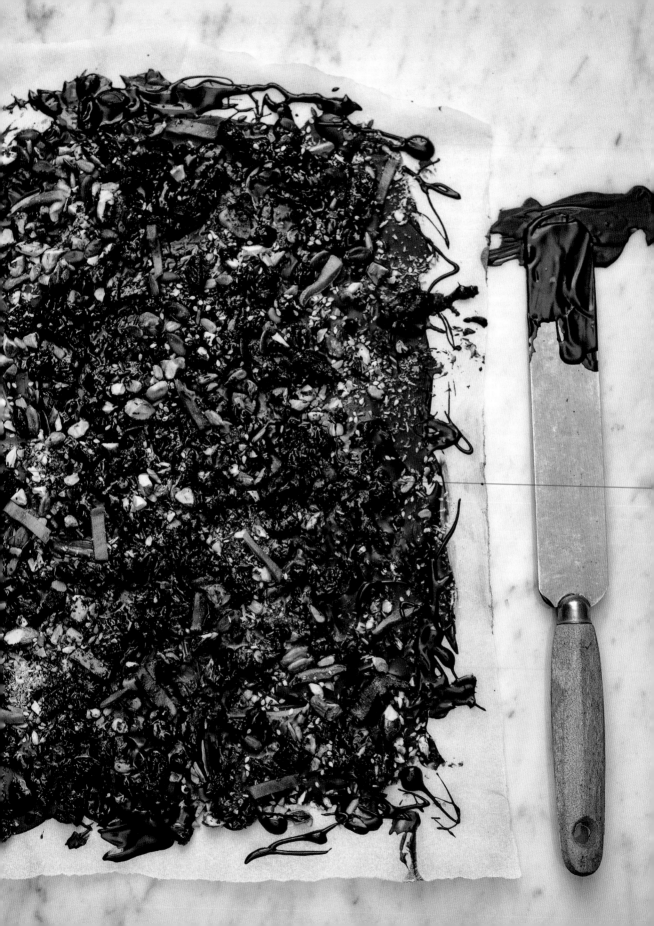

chocolate, coconut & mango thins

Prep time:
**5 minutes (plus
30 minutes chilling)**

Cooking time:
5–8 minutes

Calories per serving:
199

The perfect not-too-naughty snack that's ridiculously easy and fun to make. Be prepared to get seriously messy – especially if you get the kids involved! My favourite thing about these is the different textures: the nuts and seeds versus the solid chocolate, and the chew versus the crunch.

serves 8

150g dark chocolate (80% cocoa solids), roughly chopped

30g desiccated coconut

25g raisins

30g shelled pistachios, roughly chopped

30g dried mango, roughly chopped

30g seeds (sunflower or pumpkin seeds work really nicely)

pinch of sea salt

1/ Line a 20 x 30cm baking tray with baking paper and set aside until needed.

2/ Fill a medium-sized saucepan three-quarters full of water and place over a medium heat. Bring to the boil, then reduce the heat to a simmer. Place a heatproof bowl on top of the saucepan to make a bain-marie, making sure that the bottom of the bowl doesn't touch the water. Add the chocolate to the bowl and allow to melt, stirring occasionally, for 5–8 minutes until completely melted. Take off the heat.

3/ Meanwhile, in a separate bowl, mix together the coconut, raisins, pistachios, mango and seeds.

4/ Add half the fruit, nut and seed mixture to the melted chocolate and stir to combine.

5/ Carefully pour the chocolate mixture onto the prepared baking tray, then scatter over the rest of the fruit, nuts and seeds. Sprinkle with sea salt and transfer to the fridge for 30 minutes to set.

6/ Once set, carefully break it up into shards and enjoy!

fruit skewers

Prep time:
5 minutes

Calories per skewer:
80

These skewers are a clever way of making fruit fun for kids (and adults, to be fair). You can use whatever kind of fruit you like – the more colourful, the better. Just make sure the grapes are cut or quartered lengthways, as they can be a choking hazard for small children.

**makes 6–8 skewers
serves 6**

4 kiwi fruits, peeled and each chopped into 8 pieces

16 red or green grapes, halved or quartered lengthways (especially if serving these to kids – whole grapes can be a choking hazard)

1 mango, peeled and chopped into 2cm chunks (or 150g pre-cut mango)

100g blueberries

1 tablespoon smooth peanut butter

10g dark chocolate (80% cocoa solids), finely grated

1/ Divide the fruit between the skewers, alternating different fruits as you go to make things interesting. If you're serving these to children, be sure to use blunt skewers, or pull the fruit off for them as you serve (with a flourish).

2/ Drizzle a little peanut butter over each skewer.

3/ Scatter over the grated chocolate so that each fruit skewer gets a dusting. Enjoy straight away.

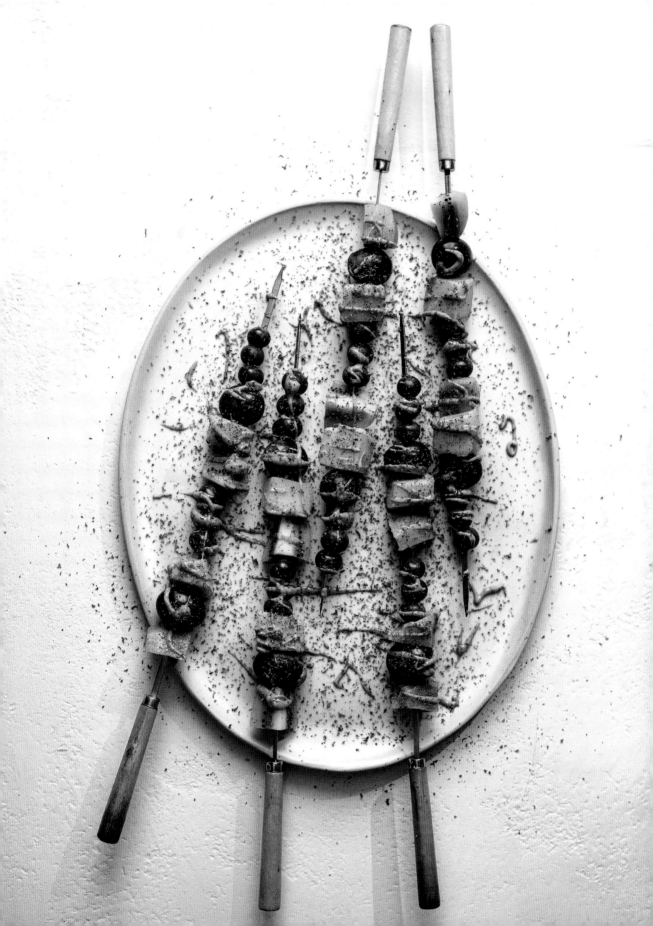

pineapple & kiwi layered pots

Prep time:
5 minutes

Calories per serving:
195

Not only are these great fun for kids to help make, they look so great you can use them as decorations instead of eating them (that's a joke – please eat them!). I've gone for pineapple and kiwi, but you can use any fruit you have lying around, including tinned (just make sure you use fruit tinned in juice, not syrup, as it's less calorific and sugary).

serves 4

400g low-fat natural yoghurt

3 kiwi fruits, peeled and sliced into rounds

1 x 227g tin pineapple slices in juice, drained and cut into bite-sized pieces

2 tablespoons nut butter (shop-bought or home-made – see page 164)

2 ginger nut biscuits, crumbled

1/ Take 4 bowls, glass ramekins or little pots, and place 1 tablespoon of the yoghurt in each. Top with a layer of kiwi fruits and pineapple, then a little nut butter, then a layer of ginger nut crumbs.

2/ Repeat the layers twice more – yoghurt, fruit, then nut butter, and always finishing with a sprinkling of ginger nut crumbs.

3/ These are great when munched immediately, but if you're making them for later, leave off the final layer of ginger nut crumbs until just before you serve.

quick tomato salsa on toast

Prep time:
5 minutes

Calories per serving:
91

I love this slathered on toast, crispbreads or oatcakes. Make sure your tomatoes are nice, juicy and ripe, as they'll have a much stronger flavour.

serves 6

500g ripe vine tomatoes

¼ small red onion

¼ garlic clove, finely grated

1 tablespoon extra-virgin olive oil

toast, oatcakes or wholemeal crackers, to serve

1/ Place the tomatoes, red onion, garlic and oil into a food-processor or blender.

2/ Pulse until combined, then spread on toast, wholemeal crackers or oatcakes and wolf down before anyone else can get their mitts on it.

butter bean hummus

Prep time:
5 minutes

Calories per serving:
176

Here, I've used butter beans rather than chickpeas to add some variety and mix things up. Butter beans are a great source of fibre and protein, but cannellini beans will also work with this recipe – as will chickpeas, of course, if you prefer to keep things classic.

serves 6

1 x 400g tin butter beans, drained

30g cashews

½ garlic clove, finely grated

2 teaspoons tahini paste

juice of 1 lemon

50ml extra-virgin olive oil

sea salt and freshly ground black pepper

1/ Place the butter beans in a blender, along with the cashews, garlic, tahini, lemon juice and oil. Season with salt and pepper and blitz to combine.

2/ Taste and adjust the seasoning if needed. Add 1 tablespoon water and blitz again. If you prefer a thinner texture, just add a little more water until you have the thickness you like.

3/ This is great served with carrot sticks or breadsticks. It will keep in the fridge in a sealed container for up to 6 days.

tomato & avocado guacamole

Prep time:
5 minutes

Calories per serving:
200

A really quick and very tasty guacamole recipe. I make up a big batch to keep in the fridge for snacking – it's great with carrot sticks or other fresh veg. You can also add a dollop of this to salads or use it as a dip for crackers. It's basically your one-stop-shop for guac (I'm a poet!).

serves 4

2 ripe avocados, peeled and stoned

3 ripe cherry vine tomatoes

2 tablespoons extra-virgin oil

juice of ½ lime, plus extra if needed

½ small red onion

sea salt and freshly ground black pepper

1/ Place all the ingredients in a blender and blend until smooth.

2/ Taste and season, adding extra lime if needed. And that's literally it. God bless blenders, right?

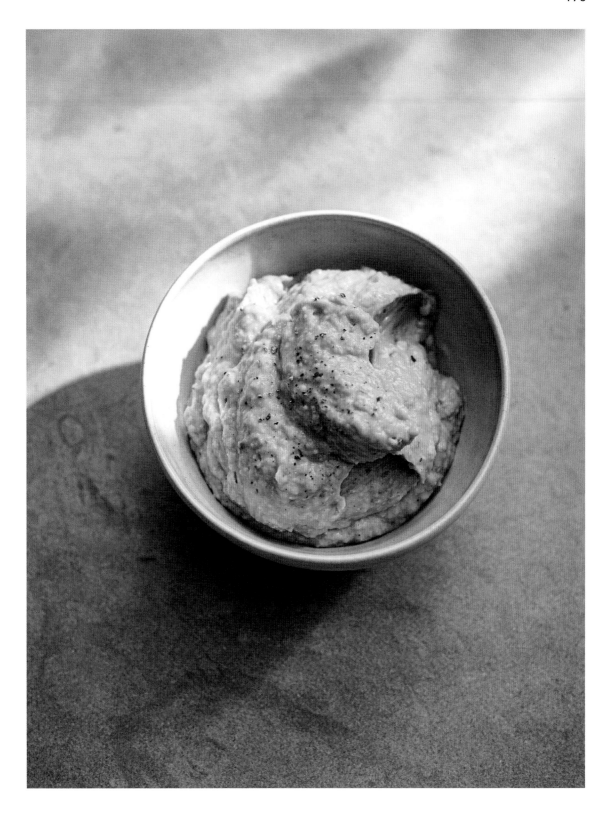

The Ultimate Body Plan for New Mums

kale crisps

Impress guests (and yourself) with these home-made kale crisps. Kale crisps are only really sold in health-food shops and can be pretty expensive, so beat the system by making your own instead. My favourite topping is sesame seeds for added crunch.

serves 4

400g kale, stalks removed

2 tablespoons olive oil

2 tablespoons sesame seeds

sea salt

1/ Preheat the oven to 200°C/180°C fan/400°F/gas 6.

2/ Place the kale in a large roasting tray. It will look like a lot of kale, but don't panic – it will really cook down!

3/ Drizzle over the olive oil and scatter over the sesame seeds. Season with a pinch of salt.

4/ Place in the oven for 10–15 minutes, until crisp, giving the tray a good shake halfway through.

5/ These kale crisps make a delicious addition to salads, and are also great as a little snack. Eat them the same day you make them.

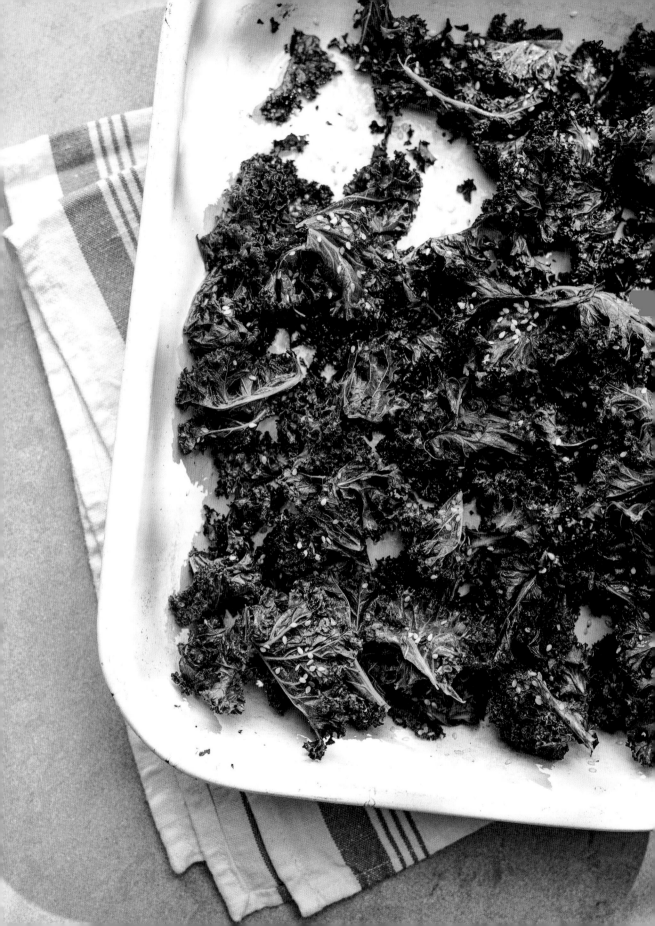

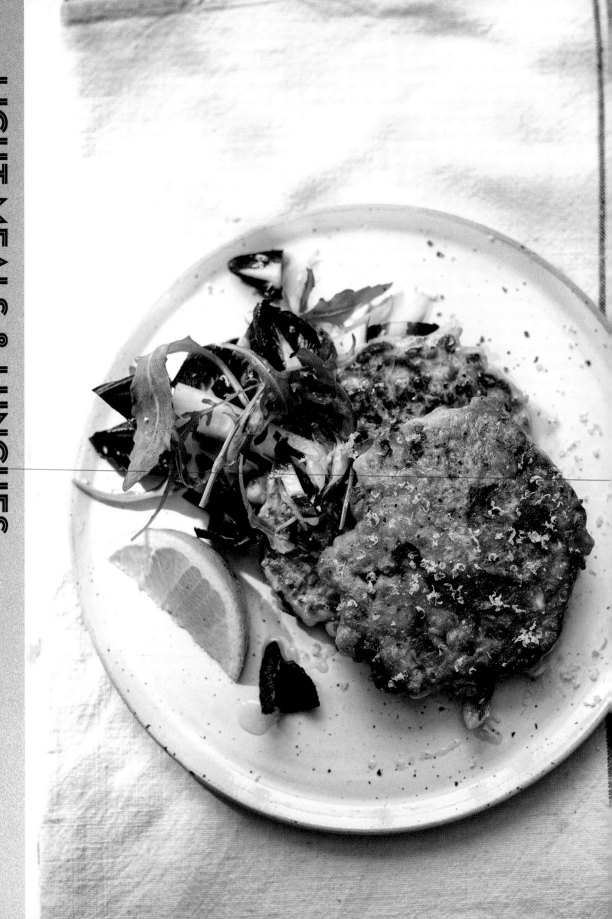

sweetcorn & spinach pancakes

Prep time:
5 minutes

Cooking time:
10 minutes

Calories per serving:
278

Kids will love to both help make and then eat these savoury pancakes. They work brilliantly using frozen sweetcorn and frozen spinach, so they're really simple to throw together. (The frozen sweetcorn can be added as is, but you need to make sure the frozen spinach is defrosted first.)

makes 8 pancakes

100g self-raising flour

1 large free-range egg

100ml unsweetened fortified oat or almond milk, or semi-skimmed cow's milk

200g frozen sweetcorn

75g fresh or frozen spinach, defrosted if using frozen, roughly chopped

50g strong vegan cheese or mature Cheddar, grated

2 sprigs of mint, leaves picked and finely chopped

sea salt and freshly ground black pepper

1 tablespoon olive oil

To serve
200g rocket and red chicory

juice of 1 lemon

1 tablespoon extra-virgin olive oil

grated Parmesan, for sprinkling (optional)

1/ In a large bowl, mix together the self-raising flour, egg and milk until well combined. Stir in the sweetcorn, spinach, cheese and mint, and season to taste.

2/ Heat the oil in a non-stick frying pan over a medium heat. Take a ladleful or a heaped tablespoon of the batter and drop into the pan. The mix makes 8 pancakes, and you should be able to cook a few at a time. Cook the pancakes for 2–3 minutes on each side until golden and cooked through. Transfer to a plate lined with kitchen paper while you cook the rest.

3/ In a salad bowl, toss together the rocket, chicory, lemon juice and oil. Serve the pancakes with the salad on the side. If you like, you can top with a sprinkling of finely grated Parmesan.

gorka's spanish omelette

This is one of Gorka's favourite dishes to make, as it reminds him of home and was the first thing his mum taught him to cook. Oh – and because it's delicious, of course! It's not quite what British people think of when they hear the word 'omelette': it's more like a flan, which makes it perfect for shared lunches, picnics or as a veggie option at a barbecue. It's great served with a tomato salad on the side.

Prep time:
10 minutes

Cooking time:
35–40 minutes

Calories per tablespoon:
599

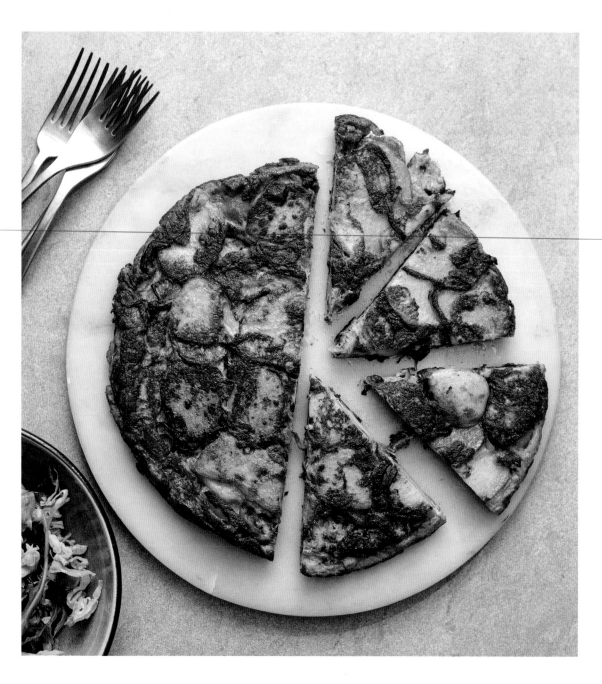

serves 6

4 large free-range eggs

splash of unsweetened fortified oat milk, or semi-skimmed cow's milk

2 tablespoons olive oil, plus extra for deep-frying

½ onion, thinly sliced

3 large potatoes (approx. 900g), peeled, quartered and thinly sliced or grated

sea salt and freshly ground black pepper

To serve
tomato and mixed leaf salad, dressed with extra-virgin olive oil and balsamic vinegar

1/ Crack the eggs into a large bowl. Add the milk and whisk to combine, then set aside.

2/ Heat 1 tablespoon of the oil in a large, deep non-stick frying pan (approx. 28–30cm in diameter) over a medium heat. Add the onion and gently fry for 5–8 minutes until softened. Remove from the pan and add to the bowl of whisked eggs.

3/ Return the pan to the heat and carefully pour in enough oil to fill the pan about a third full. Wait until the oil is heated through. You can test this by dropping in a little piece of potato – if the oil starts to bubble around it, it's good to go.

4/ You will need to fry the potatoes in 2 batches to be safe. Add half the potatoes to the pan, making sure the oil is covering them. Cook for 10 minutes, or until the potatoes are soft.

5/ Line a colander with some kitchen paper, then use a slotted spoon to remove the cooked potatoes from the pan and dab off any excess oil. Repeat with the remaining potatoes.

6/ Place the cooked potatoes in the bowl with the eggs and onion and mix to combine. Season with a little salt and pepper.

7/ Heat the remaining 1 tablespoon of oil in another large non-stick frying pan over a low heat. Pour the contents of the bowl into the frying pan and cook for 5 minutes. At first, move the spoon through the middle of the pan a few times to help cook the middle of the omelette, then leave it alone. As it cooks, use a fish slice to ease the edges of the omelette away from the sides of the pan, giving the pan the occasional shake to make sure it is not catching on the bottom. When the bottom of the omelette is no longer sticking to the bottom of pan, it's time to flip.

8/ Place a large plate on top of the pan, then carefully but firmly flip the pan over and twist the plate underneath. This should release the omelette onto the plate.

9/ Slide the omelette back into the pan, cooked-side up, and fry for a further 2–3 minutes to cook the other side.

10/ Remove the omelette from the pan and cut into wedges. Serve with a lovely big balsamic-dressed salad on the side.

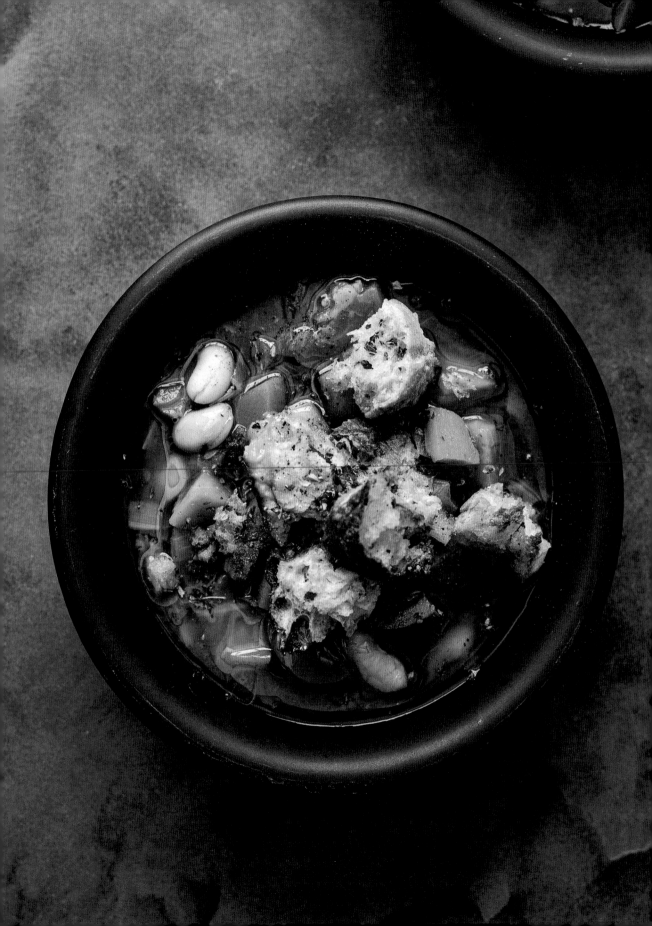

chunky veg soup

Ahh, veg prep – the bane of any cook's life. My solution: whack on some music or a podcast and zone out as you chop! I actually find it really relaxing. And this recipe is so worth it, because once all that chopping's done, all you have to do is stir and then leave well alone. This soup is perfect for freezing and reheating. Top with some freshly baked torn ciabatta for added texture (and flair).

Prep time:
8–10 minutes (depending on your chopping skills!)

Cooking time:
30–40 minutes

Calories per serving:
372

serves 6

250g ciabatta, torn into bite-sized pieces

2 tablespoons dried herbs (I like to use oregano or mixed herbs)

2 tablespoons olive oil

1 onion, finely chopped

2 carrots, roughly chopped into 2cm chunks

2 celery sticks, trimmed and chopped into 2cm chunks

1 leek, halved lengthways and sliced

1 courgette, trimmed, quartered lengthways, and chopped into 2cm chunks

1 large sweet potato, peeled and chopped into 2cm chunks

2 tablespoons tomato purée

2¼ pints vegetable stock

1 x 400g tin butter beans, drained

sea salt and freshly ground black pepper

1/ Preheat the oven to 200°C/180°C fan/400°F/gas 6.

2/ Place the torn ciabatta on a baking tray. Sprinkle over 1 tablespoon of the dried herbs and drizzle with 1 tablespoon of the oil. Toss to coat, then bake for 10–15 minutes or until golden and crisp. Remove from the oven and set aside for later.

3/ Heat the remaining 1 tablespoon olive oil in a large non-stick saucepan over a medium heat.

4/ Add the onion, carrots, celery, leek and courgette and cook for 10–15 minutes, stirring occasionally.

5/ Once these are softened and getting nice and golden, add the sweet potato, tomato purée and remaining dried herbs. Give it all a good stir, then pour in the stock and cook for 10 minutes, uncovered, until the sweet potato is cooked through. Add the beans and stir to warm through, then season to taste.

6/ Serve in bowls, and top each one with a handful of herby torn ciabatta – a fancy version of croutons.

pumpkin or butternut squash soup

Prep time:
8 minutes

Cooking time:
45 minutes

Calories per serving:
239

If you make this during the autumn, please use pumpkin, as it's so damn good. While you may be tempted to chop up the leftover jack-o'-lanterns your kids have 'carved' (read: destroyed) and create something delicious out of the wreckage, I recommend choosing some pumpkins from the food aisle of your local supermarket instead. They'll be much tastier. If it's not the season, butternut squash is the perfect alternative. (Please note: you do peel the pumpkin, but you don't peel the squash).

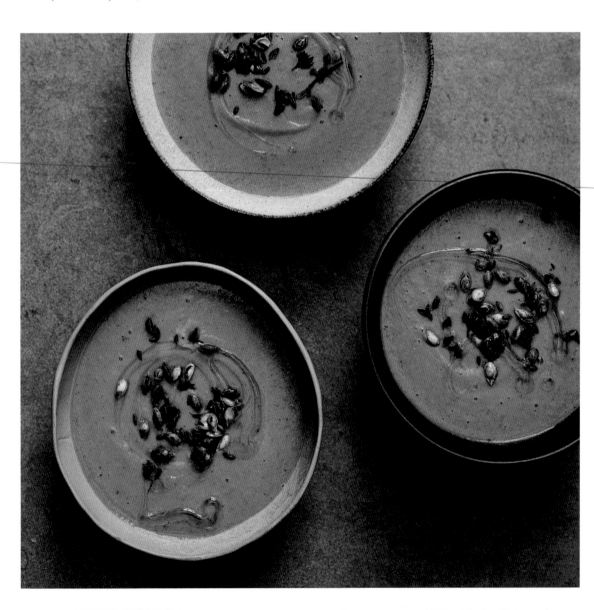

serves 6

1 pumpkin or butternut squash (approx. 900g)

3 tablespoons olive oil

generous pinch of ground cinnamon

sea salt and freshly ground black pepper

2 garlic cloves, roughly chopped

1 large onion, roughly chopped

1 small fennel bulb, roughly chopped

4–5 sprigs of thyme

1¾ pints vegetable stock

1 x 400g tin light coconut milk

150g dried red lentils

1 tablespoon fennel seeds

1/ Preheat the oven to 220°C/200°C fan/425°F/gas 7.

2/ If you're using a pumpkin, peel the skin (there is no need to peel a butternut squash). Roughly chop the pumpkin or squash into 2cm pieces, removing the seeds and setting them aside for later.

3/ Place the chunks of pumpkin or squash on a large roasting tray. Drizzle over 1 tablespoon of the olive oil, and sprinkle over the cinnamon, along with some salt and black pepper. Toss together to coat, then cover with tin foil. Roast for 20 minutes, then remove the foil and roast, uncovered, for a further 10 minutes.

4/ Meanwhile, heat 1 tablespoon of the oil in a large non-stick saucepan over a medium heat. Add the garlic, onion, fennel bulb and thyme sprigs, and cook for 10–15 minutes or until soft and a little golden.

5/ Add the stock, coconut milk and lentils, and cook for a further 25 minutes, or until the lentils are cooked through and the soup is thickening up. Pick out the thyme sprigs and pull off the leaves. Return the leaves to the soup and discard the twigs.

6/ Once the butternut squash or pumpkin has finished roasting, add it to the soup, but leave the oven on. You can keep the soup chunky, if you like, or you can transfer it to a blender or use a hand-held blender to blitz until smooth. I like to blitz about half the soup in a blender and then stir it back through. If you prefer a thinner soup, you can add more stock or some hot water. Keep the soup warm while you prepare the seeds.

7/ Wash the pumpkin or squash seeds and pat them dry using kitchen paper, then place them in the same roasting tray you used to roast the squash or pumpkin. Drizzle over the remaining 1 tablespoon olive oil and sprinkle over the fennel seeds. Toss to combine, then roast for 5 minutes or until golden and crispy.

8/ Serve the soup in bowls, topped with the roasted seeds.

veggie shepherd's pie

Prep time:
5–10 minutes

Cooking time:
1 hour 25 minutes

Calories per serving
(of shepherd's pie):
313

You'll see in the ingredient list that most of the veg used here needs to be 'roughly chopped' before being pulsed in the food-processor, which is a result, as it means your food-processor can do the hard work for you. Just chuck it in and breathe a sigh of relief. This recipe makes more than you need for the pie, so you should have a batch of 4 servings of sauce leftover that you can either freeze or use in other dishes (for example, as a baked potato filling or to stir through cooked pasta).

serves 6
(plus makes an extra batch of lentil mix, for freezing)

1 large onion, roughly chopped

2 carrots, roughly chopped

2 celery sticks, roughly chopped

1 fennel bulb, roughly chopped

1 tablespoon olive oil

2 garlic cloves, finely chopped

2 sprigs of rosemary, finely chopped, or 1 teaspoon dried rosemary

2 tablespoons tomato purée

2 x 400g tins chopped tomatoes

250g dried red lentils

1 tablespoon balsamic vinegar

sea salt and freshly ground black pepper

400g potatoes, peeled and chopped

400g sweet potatoes, peeled and chopped

30g unsalted butter

20g mature Cheddar, grated

1/ Place the onion, carrots, celery and fennel into a food-processor and pulse 3–4 times to finely chop without turning it all into mush.

2/ Heat the oil in a large saucepan over a medium heat. Add the garlic and rosemary, along with the mixture from the food-processor. Sweat for 10–15 minutes, stirring occasionally.

3/ Once everything is cooked and softened, add the tomato purée and stir to combine, then add the tinned tomatoes. Fill up both tins with water, swirl and pour into the pan, then half-fill one of the tins with water once more, and add that, too. Stir in the lentils. Reduce the heat to medium–low and let it simmer away for 40–50 minutes until the lentils are cooked. Stir in the balsamic vinegar, then season to taste with salt and pepper.

4/ Meanwhile, preheat the oven to 200°C/180°C fan/400°F/gas 6. Bring a separate large saucepan of water to the boil. Add the white potatoes and cook for 5 minutes, then add the sweet potatoes and cook for a further 10 minutes. Drain and leave to steam before mashing with a little butter.

5/ Put 1.5kg of the lentil mix into a 20 x 30cm ovenproof dish. Top with the mashed potatoes, then sprinkle over the grated Cheddar and bake for 20 minutes until golden and bubbling.

6/ The remaining lentil mix will keep in the fridge in an airtight container for 3–5 days, or in the freezer for up to 3 months. It's perfect with a jacket potato, stirred though pasta or served with chipolatas or veggie sausages.

fish finger wraps with crunchy salad

Prep time:
5 minutes

Cooking time:
15 minutes

Calories per serving:
433

A fancier (and healthier) version of every 1990s kid's favourite snack. Try to use wholemeal wraps if you can, and make a huge amount of the salad as it goes brilliantly with other dishes, too. I recommend using it in a pitta with some poached salmon or grilled chicken.

serves 4

8 good-quality sustainably sourced fish fingers

100g Little Gem or iceberg lettuce, shredded

180g red cabbage, shredded

100g cucumber, finely diced

10 cherry tomatoes, finely diced

2 tablespoons Greek yoghurt

2 tablespoons capers

handful of dill, finely chopped

1 tablespoon extra-virgin olive oil

sea salt and freshly ground black pepper

4 large wholemeal wraps

4–6 teaspoons tomato ketchup

1/ Preheat the oven and cook the fish fingers according to the packet instructions.

2/ Meanwhile, put the shredded lettuce and cabbage into a bowl, then stir in the diced cucumber and tomatoes. Add the yoghurt, capers, dill and extra-virgin olive oil and season with salt and pepper.

3/ To make up the wraps, spread each one with some tomato ketchup, then add 2 fish fingers to each wrap. Top with the slaw-style salad, roll up and enjoy!

sesame soba noodle bowl

Prep time:
15 minutes

Cooking time:
15 minutes

Calories per serving:
600

A tasty and healthy dish that can be eaten either hot or cold.
Add a soft-boiled egg on top and some chilli sauce for that proper
Asian twist.

serves 4

200g dried soba noodles

300g red cabbage, finely shredded

1 tablespoon sesame oil

4 salmon fillets (approx. 120g each), skin on

125g sugar snap peas, halved lengthways

bunch of spring onions, trimmed and finely chopped

125g fresh or frozen edamame beans, defrosted if frozen

2 tablespoons chilli sauce, to serve (optional)

For the dressing
2 tablespoons sesame seeds, toasted

1 tablespoon sesame oil

3 tablespoons low-salt soy sauce

1 teaspoon runny honey

juice of 1 lime

1 garlic clove, finely grated

1/ Cook your noodles according to the packet instructions. Drain, then give them a good rinse in cold water and set aside.

2/ To make the dressing, combine all the dressing ingredients in a large bowl. Add the shredded cabbage and give it a good scrunch to combine, then set aside.

3/ Heat the sesame oil in a large non-stick frying pan over a high heat. Add the salmon fillets, skin-side down. Cook for 12 minutes, turning halfway through. Add the sugar snap peas to the pan for the final 4 minutes. Remove the salmon and peas from the pan and set aside.

4/ Add the drained noodles, spring onions and edamame beans to the cabbage in the bowl and give it all a good mix to combine. Drizzle over the chilli sauce, if using.

5/ Serve topped with the salmon fillets and sugar snap peas, and marvel at how beautiful it all looks before getting stuck in.

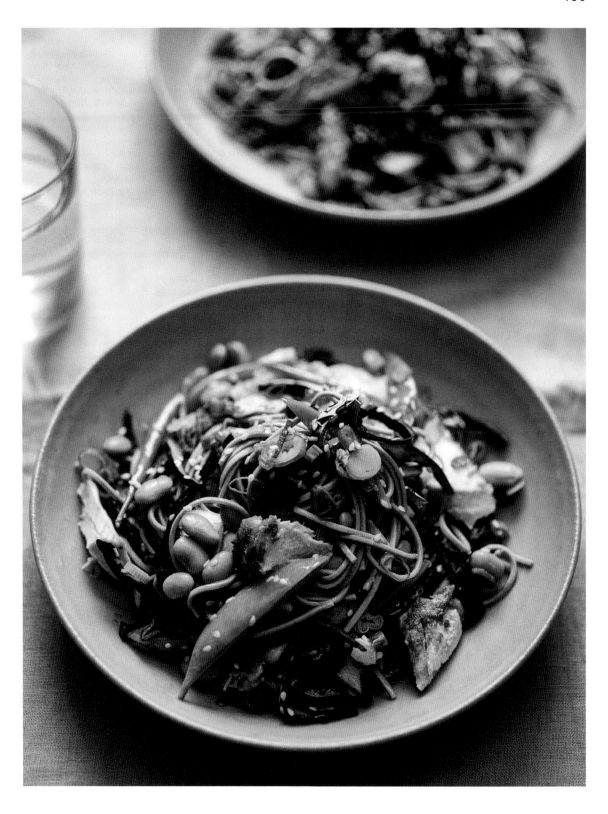

The Ultimate Body Plan for New Mums

ginger & sesame pan-seared tuna with lentils

Prep time:
5 minutes

Cooking time:
5 minutes

Calories per serving:
563

One to impress the neighbours, this! A proper 'wow' dish. I always keep a couple of pouches of lentils in the cupboard for those days when I'm after a filling but speedy addition to my lunch. And it's worth a trip to the fishmongers or supermarket fish counter to splash out on some really lovely tuna fillets if you can.

serves 2

3cm piece of fresh root ginger, grated

1 heaped tablespoon sesame seeds

sea salt and freshly ground black pepper

2 tablespoons sesame oil

2 fresh, sustainably sourced yellowfin tuna steaks (approx. 120g each)

3 tablespoons reduced-salt soy sauce

3 tablespoons rice wine vinegar

juice of 1 lime

250g pouch precooked Puy lentils

500g greens of your choice (I used 300g pak choi and 200g sugar snap peas)

1/ In a small bowl, mix together the ginger, sesame seeds, a good pinch of black pepper and 1 tablespoon of the sesame oil.

2/ Place the tuna steaks on a board and rub the ginger mix onto them, along with a little sea salt.

3/ In another bowl, mix together the soy sauce, rice wine vinegar and lime juice and set aside.

4/ Place a large non-stick frying pan over a high heat and sear the tuna steaks for 1 minute on each side, then set them aside on a plate to rest. (As long as the tuna is good quality and fresh, just searing it like this is totally safe.)

5/ Keep the pan on the heat and add the remaining 1 tablespoon sesame oil. Add the lentils and greens and stir-fry for a couple of minutes, then pour over half the soy sauce mixture and stir to combine.

6/ Divide the lentils and greens between 2 plates. Slice the tuna steaks on an angle and arrange on top of the lentils, then pour over the remaining sauce and serve.

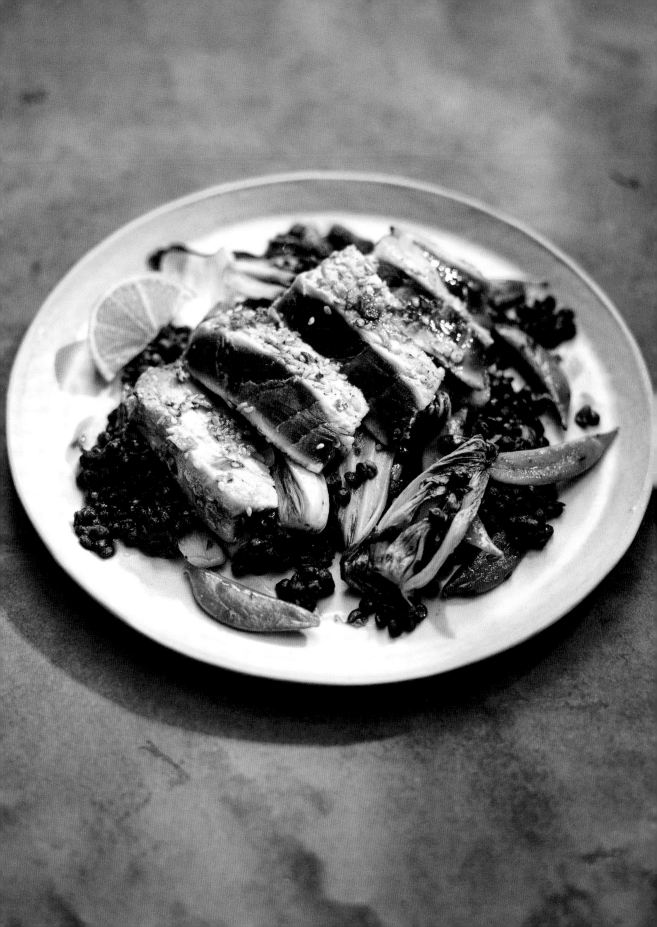

tuna, tomato & caper pasta

Prep time:
5 minutes

Cooking time:
15 minutes

Calories per serving:
317

A fresh-tasting, last-minute meal that will fill you up. Try to buy tuna in spring water, not brine (it's healthier and less salty), and also look for the MSC (Marine Stewardship Council) blue fish label. This means the tuna is certified as traceable and sustainable. I use wholemeal pasta as it contains more fibre than traditional pasta made from durum wheat, and it fills you up for longer.

serves 4

1 tablespoon sea salt

250g wholemeal penne (or other pasta shape of your choice)

1 tablespoon olive oil

2 garlic cloves, finely chopped or crushed

2 heaped tablespoons capers

300g cherry vine tomatoes, halved

2 x 160g tins sustainably sourced tuna in spring water, drained

zest and juice of 1 lemon

few handfuls of rocket

sea salt and freshly ground black pepper

1/ Add the 1 tablespoon of sea salt to a large saucepan filled with water and bring to the boil.

2/ Add the pasta and cook for 10 minutes (or according to the packet instructions).

3/ Meanwhile, heat the oil in a large non-stick saucepan over a medium heat and add the garlic, capers and tomatoes. Cook for 5 minutes, adding a splash of water at the end if the mixture seems too thick.

4/ Stir in the tuna and lemon zest and juice, and simmer for a further 5 minutes.

5/ Once the pasta is done, drain, reserving about a cupful of the pasta water. Add the cooked pasta to the pan of sauce along with most of the reserved pasta water (you can add more if needed), then stir through the rocket until it wilts.

6/ Taste and season before serving.

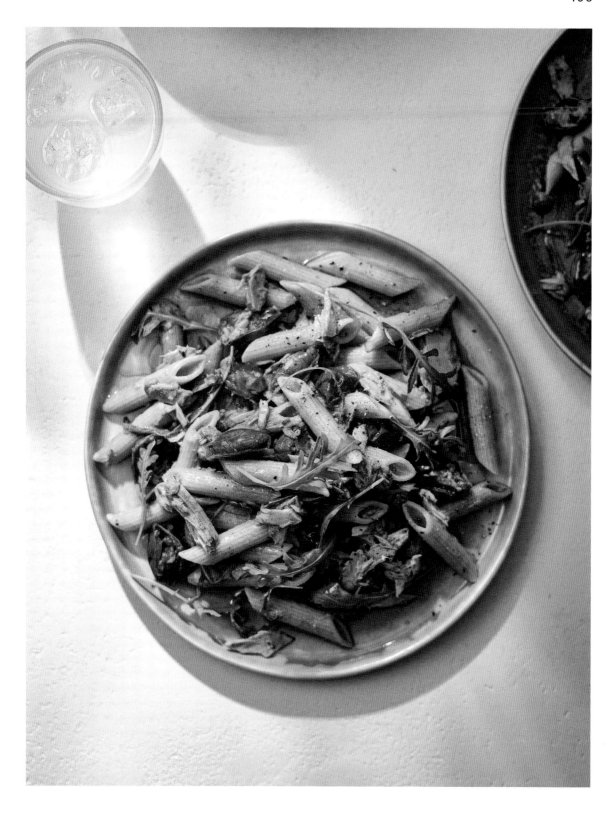

The Ultimate Body Plan for New Mums

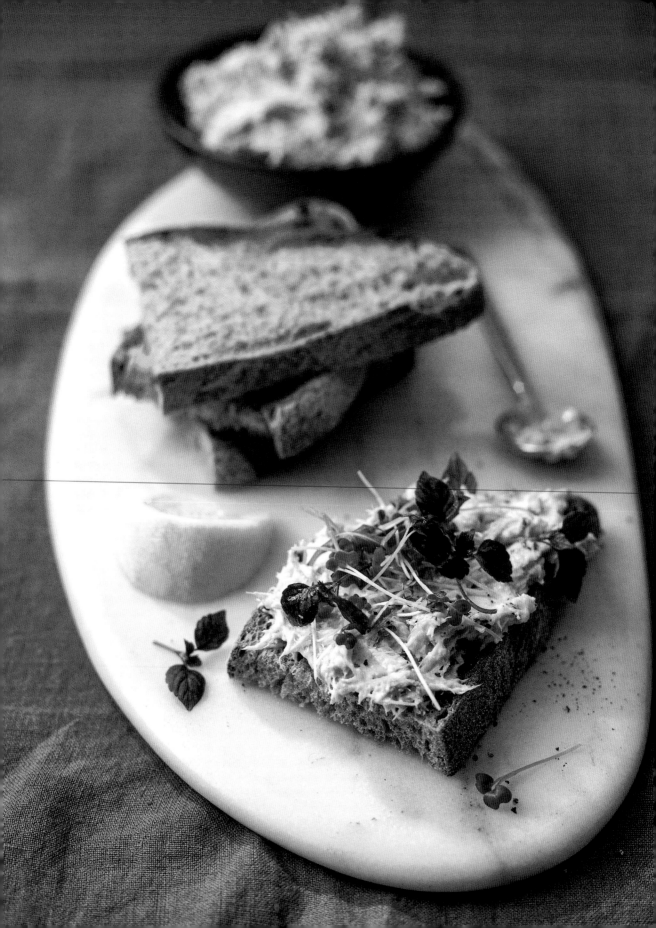

quick smoked mackerel pâté

Prep time:
5 minutes

Calories per serving:
280

Making your own pâté is super impressive when you have guests over, and this version tastes incredible. It's light in flavour and, as this recipe uses precooked mackerel, the fish requires no prep. Mackerel is an oily fish and so contains omega-3 (see page 139). Please note: breastfeeding mums shouldn't consume more than two portions of oily fish per week.

serves 4

180g sustainably sourced smoked mackerel fillets, skin removed

3 tablespoons Greek yoghurt

zest and juice of 1 lemon

½ small bunch of chives, finely chopped

sea salt and freshly ground black pepper

To serve
4 slices of wholemeal bread

handful of cress, mini salad leaves, watercress or rocket

extra-virgin olive oil and balsamic vinegar, for dressing

1/ Place the mackerel in a bowl with the yoghurt and lemon zest and juice. Mix together until the mackerel fillets break down and form a paste and everything is well combined.

2/ Add the chives and stir again, seasoning to taste.

3/ Toast the bread and slice the pieces of toast in half. Dress your chosen salad leaves with the olive oil and vinegar. Spread the mackerel pâté on the hot toast, then serve with the salad leaves on the side or scattered over the top.

crispy katsu chicken lettuce cups

Prep time:
10 minutes

Cooking time:
6–8 minutes

Calories per serving:
350

There's a lot to love about this dish: the strong katsu curry flavour works beautifully with the crunchy, tender chicken, the lettuce cups provide a satisfying textural contrast, and you don't need any additional rice or pasta to fill you up. Perfect.

serves 4

2 skinless free-range chicken breasts (approx. 335g total weight)

65g stale wholemeal bread

1 garlic clove

small bunch of thyme, leaves picked

3 tablespoons olive oil

2 tablespoons plain flour

1 teaspoon mild curry powder

1 large free-range egg

2 carrots, grated

1 large courgette, grated

sea salt and freshly ground black pepper

2–3 Little Gem lettuces, trimmed and leaves separated

½ cucumber, cut into matchsticks

4 heaped tablespoons natural yoghurt

2 tablespoons sweet chilli sauce (optional)

fresh red chilli slices, to serve

1/ Place the chicken breasts between two sheets of baking paper, then bash with a flat-bottomed saucepan to flatten them out to a thickness of about 0.5cm.

2/ Place the bread, garlic and thyme in a small blender with 1 tablespoon of the olive oil. Blitz to create flavoured breadcrumbs, then pour into a shallow bowl and set aside.

3/ Take out 2 more shallow bowls. In one, mix together the flour and curry powder. In the other, whisk the egg.

4/ In a large bowl, mix together the carrots and courgette and drizzle with 1 tablespoon of the olive oil. Season and set aside.

5/ Take one of the flattened chicken breasts and dip it into the flavoured flour, then the egg, moving it about to make sure it is fully coated. Let any excess drip off, then dip it in the breadcrumbs, turning to coat well, making sure the chicken is completely covered. Repeat with the second chicken breast.

6/ Heat the remaining 1 tablespoon oil in a medium-sized frying pan over a medium–high heat. Add the chicken and cook for 3–4 minutes on each side until it's cooked through and the breadcrumbs are nice and golden. Remove from the pan and set aside on a plate lined with kitchen paper to rest.

7/ To serve, slice the chicken on an angle to create strips, then lay out all your remaining ingredients. For each cup, take a lettuce leaf and add a little of the carrot and courgette salad. Top with some sliced chicken, cucumber, a little yoghurt, a drizzle of sweet chilli sauce (if using) and some fresh chilli slices.

roasted sweet potatoes with hummus and greens

Prep time:
5 minutes

Cooking time:
1 hour

Calories per serving:
527

A properly comforting dish that can be topped with anything you fancy. For me that means hummus (home-made! See page 173), loads of greens and a generous sprinkle of toasted seeds. If you're a meat-eater, I'd recommend doing what Gorka does for him and Mia: frying up a little chorizo and throwing that on, too.

serves 4

4 sweet potatoes, washed

3 tablespoons olive oil

sea salt and freshly ground black pepper

350g mixed greens (I like to use kale, rainbow chard and spring greens), trimmed and roughly chopped

juice of ½ lemon

4 heaped tablespoons hummus (home-made, see page 173, or shop-bought)

4 tablespoons soured cream or natural yoghurt

4 tablespoons mixed seeds, toasted

1/ Preheat the oven to 200°C/180°C fan/400°F/gas 6.

2/ Use a fork to prick the sweet potatoes all over, then place in a snug-fitting roasting tray and rub with 2 tablespoons of the olive oil. Season with salt and pepper.

3/ Place in the oven and bake for 1 hour, turning halfway through, or until soft and golden – keep an eye on them to make sure they don't burn.

4/ Meanwhile, to cook your greens, place a large saucepan over a medium heat and add the remaining 1 tablespoon oil and a splash of water. Add the greens and cook for 5 minutes, stirring occasionally. At the end of the cooking time, stir in the lemon juice and season with salt and pepper.

5/ Serve the baked sweet potatoes topped with the hummus and greens, along with a dollop of soured cream or yoghurt and a scattering of mixed seeds.

black bean goodness bowl

Prep time:
10 minutes

Cooking time:
30 minutes

Calories per serving:
600

This big old bowl of healthy deliciousness can give birth to lots of other dishes, too: any leftover walnut pesto can be used as a snacking dip for veggies, while the black beans make a perfect jacket potato filling with crumbled feta and salad on the side.

serves 4

½ head of cauliflower (approx. 300g), chopped into bite-sized florets and stalk finely chopped

2 tablespoons olive oil

sea salt and black pepper

250g brown rice (or use 2 x 250g pouches brown microwave rice)

1 teaspoon smoked paprika

6 spring onions, trimmed and roughly chopped

1 x 400g tin black beans, drained

2 handfuls of fresh spinach

1 ripe avocado, peeled, stoned and sliced

20g feta cheese, crumbled

For the quick pickled onion
½ small red onion, finely sliced

1 teaspoon golden caster sugar

2 tablespoons red wine vinegar

pinch of sea salt

For the pesto
150g broccoli florets

30g walnuts, toasted

½ garlic clove, peeled

2 tablespoons extra-virgin olive oil

20g Parmesan, grated

zest and juice of ½ lemon

1/ Preheat the oven to 200°C/180°C fan/400°F/gas 6. Spread out the cauliflower on a baking tray. Sprinkle over a little water and 1 tablespoon of the olive oil. Season, then roast for 30 minutes.

2/ If you're using dried rice, cook according to the packet instructions. (If you're using microwave rice, prepare it later.)

3/ Meanwhile, place all the quick pickled onion ingredients in a bowl. Scrunch it all together until it is well mixed and the onion is beginning to soften. Stir in 2 tablespoons water and set aside.

4/ For the pesto, bring a medium-sized pan of salted water to the boil. Add the broccoli and cook for 5 minutes, then drain and add to a blender, along with the walnuts, garlic, extra-virgin olive oil, Parmesan and lemon zest and juice. Add a splash of water, then whizz to combine into a paste. Taste and season, adding a little more lemon juice if needed. Set aside.

5/ Heat the remaining 1 tablespoon oil in a small saucepan over a medium heat and add the smoked paprika and all but a small handful of the spring onions. Cook for 3 minutes, stirring, then add the black beans. Increase the heat to high and cook for 8–10 minutes until thick, stirring constantly. Season.

6/ If you're using microwave rice, prepare it now. Pour the cooked rice into a large bowl and stir in half the pesto. Place the spinach in a colander and pour over some boiling water to wilt.

7/ To assemble, divide the rice between 4 serving bowls and top with the black beans, roasted cauliflower and wilted spinach. Now scatter over the avocado, feta and quick pickled onions, and finish with a dollop of the leftover pesto and the reserved spring onions. There you have it: a bowl of goodness.

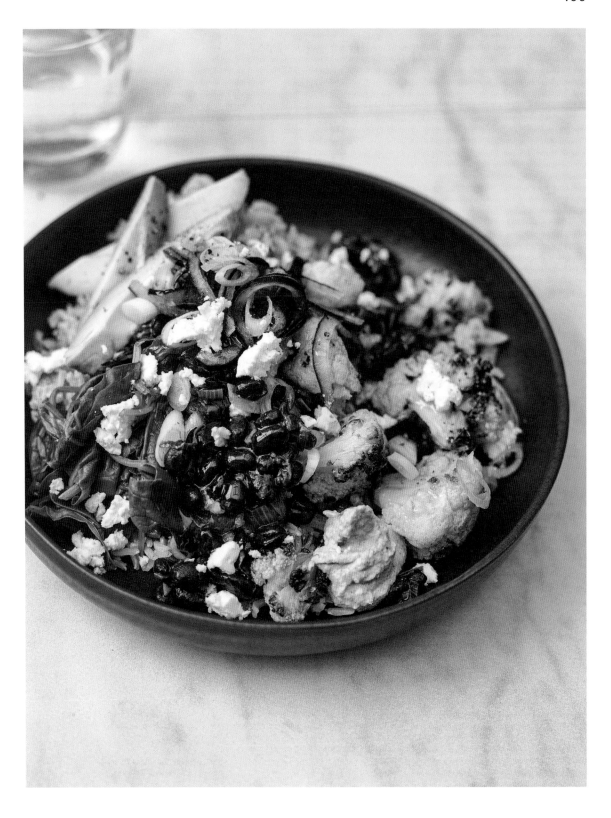

The Ultimate Body Plan for New Mums

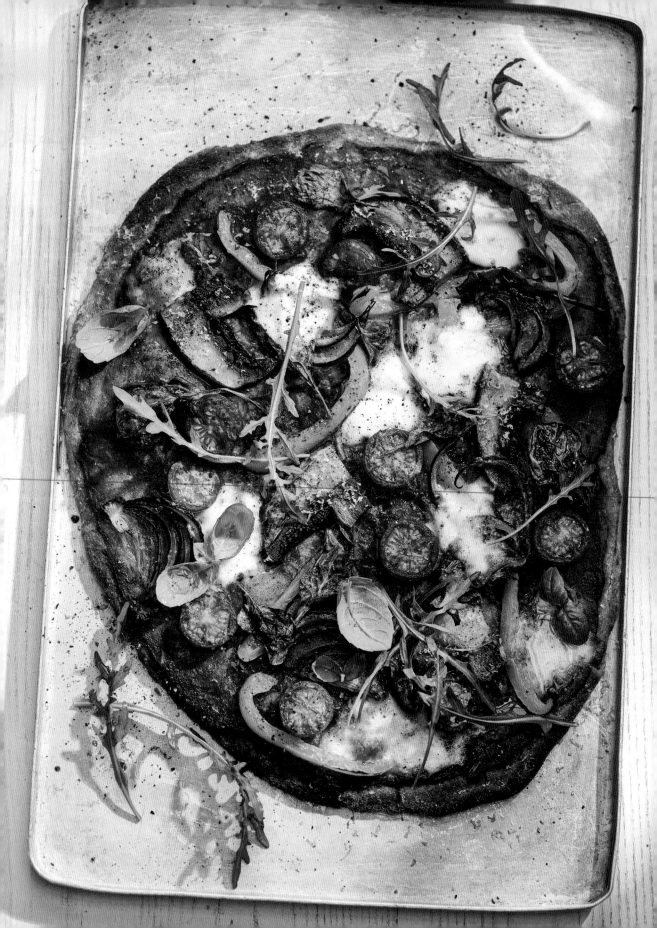

wholemeal flatbread pizzas

Prep time:
20–25 minutes

Cooking time:
8 minutes

Calories per serving:
527

This pizza dough is incredibly simple to make and it also freezes really well, so you can part-bake the bases (just roll them out, don't top them, and bake for 3–4 minutes), then freeze them to use another time (you can bake them from frozen). If you can't be bothered to make a base at all, simply buy a wholemeal flatbread from the supermarket and top with the sauce and veg – a quick cheat for a healthy pizza.

makes 2 x 25cm pizzas
serves 4

For the topping

1 small yellow or red pepper, cut into strips

1 small red onion, cut into thin wedges

100g mushrooms, sliced

8 ripe cherry tomatoes, halved

sea salt and black pepper

1 tablespoon olive oil

150g mozzarella (or a vegan cheese alternative), torn

30g spinach or rocket

handful of grated Parmesan

For the dough

300g wholemeal self-raising flour, plus extra for dusting

1 heaped teaspoon baking powder

pinch of sea salt

300g natural or Greek yoghurt

2 tablespoons olive oil

For the sauce

½ x 400g tin plum tomatoes

½ small bunch of basil, leaves picked

1 garlic clove, peeled

splash of extra-virgin olive oil

1/ Preheat the oven to its highest possible temperature (if you have a combined oven and grill, use the grill setting and preheat to high). Place 2 large baking trays in the oven to preheat.

2/ To prepare the topping ingredients, place the red pepper, onion, mushrooms and cherry tomatoes in a large bowl. Season with salt and pepper, drizzle over the oil and set aside.

3/ For the pizza dough, combine the flour, baking powder, salt, yoghurt and olive oil in a large bowl. Mix until it forms a ball, then knead for a few minutes on a floured surface until smooth.

4/ To make the tomato sauce, place the tomatoes in a blender with the basil stalks, garlic and extra-virgin olive oil, and blitz to combine.

5/ Divide the dough into 2 evenly sized balls, then use a rolling pin to roll them out into rough circles approx. 25cm in diameter.

6/ Carefully remove the preheated baking trays from the oven and place on a heatproof surface. Place the pizza bases on the trays and add half the sauce to each, spreading it out over the bases and leaving a 1cm gap around the edges.

7/ Top each pizza with half of the prepared vegetables and mozzarella, then place in the oven and bake for 8 minutes.

8/ Carefully remove the pizzas from the oven. Top with the basil leaves and spinach or rocket, along with a grating of Parmesan, and serve. (If you only have one baking tray, prepare the pizzas one after the other and eat as you go!)

halloumi pittas

Prep time:
10 minutes

Cooking time:
8–10 minutes

Calories per serving:
474

Halloumi pittas are one of my go-to dishes when I want a super-satisfying yet simple lunch. The soft yet crispy halloumi combined with loads of lovely fresh salad is always a winner, and the wholemeal pittas add extra flavour and fibre.

serves 6

1 heaped tablespoon dried oregano

1 garlic clove, finely chopped or crushed

1 tablespoon red wine vinegar

a good squeeze of lemon

400g halloumi, drained and cut into 2cm slices

1 red onion, cut into thin wedges

½ cucumber, de-seeded and grated

200g Greek yoghurt

handful of mint leaves, finely chopped

sea salt and freshly ground black pepper

6 round wholemeal pitta breads, if you can get them (or standard wholemeal pittas)

4 Little Gem lettuces or ½ cos lettuce, trimmed and shredded

handful of cherry tomatoes, halved

1/ Preheat the oven to 220°C/200°C fan/400°F/gas 7 and line a baking tray with baking paper.

2/ In a bowl, mix together the dried oregano, garlic, red wine vinegar and lemon juice. Add the halloumi and onion and give it a good mix, leaving to one side to marinate while you prepare the tzatziki.

3/ Place the grated cucumber in a bowl and stir in the yoghurt and mint. Season with salt and pepper.

4/ Add the halloumi and onion to the prepared baking tray and bake for 8–10 minutes, turning halfway through.

5/ Add the pitta breads to the oven for the last few minutes to warm through.

6/ To assemble, spread the inside of each pitta with a little tzatziki, then add some lettuce, halloumi and cherry tomatoes. Serve straight away.

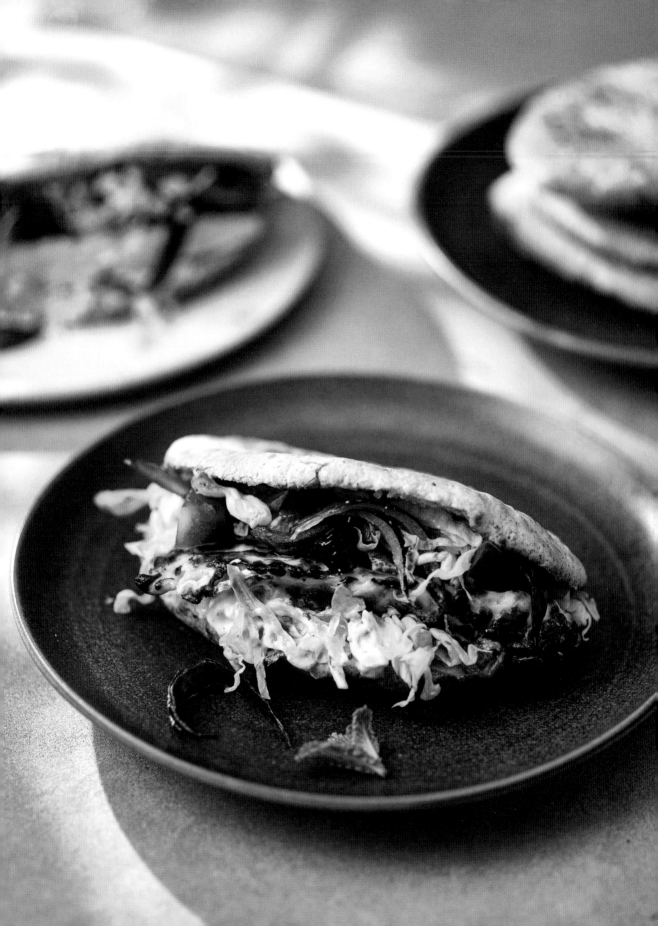

salmon & greens filo tart

Prep time:
10 minutes

Cooking time:
50–55 minutes

Calories per serving:
336

Making a tart from scratch may sound like a drag, but it's actually really easy and a lot of fun. I use whatever green veg I have in the freezer – broccoli, spinach, kale or peas all work. And, while dill is a great addition, you can swap it for chives, mint or some flat-leaf parsley.

serves 8

1 tablespoon olive oil, plus extra for brushing

3 garlic cloves, crushed

300g spring greens, trimmed and stalks removed, roughly chopped

250g fresh or frozen green beans

6 large free-range eggs

2 x 170g tins sustainably sourced salmon fillets, drained

300g cottage cheese

small bunch of dill, roughly chopped

30g mature Cheddar, grated

sea salt and freshly ground black pepper

270g shop-bought filo pastry

To serve

250g vine tomatoes, halved

½ cucumber, roughly chopped

extra-virgin olive oil and balsamic vinegar, for drizzling

1/ Preheat the oven to 210°C/190°C fan/410°F/gas 6½. Heat the oil in a 26cm ovenproof shallow frying pan over a medium–high heat. Add the garlic, spring greens and green beans and cook for 10 minutes, stirring occasionally.

2/ Crack the eggs into a large bowl and mix in the salmon, cottage cheese, dill and Cheddar. Season generously.

3/ Add the cooked greens and beans to the bowl, then give the pan a little wipe – you will use this to cook your tart.

4/ Take a large piece of baking paper and scrunch it up, then hold it under running water and keep scrunching. This makes it more flexible and helps it hold its shape better.

5/ Use this piece of baking paper to line the pan. Take out a few sheets of filo pastry and lay them in the pan, overlapping one another so that you create a full layer of pastry with edges hanging over the sides. Brush with a little oil, then repeat this process until all the filo is used up.

6/ Pour the salmon and greens mixture into the pastry-lined pan, then fold the overhanging pastry into the middle to create a pie.

7/ Bake in the middle of the oven for 40–45 minutes, or until golden and cooked through. Remove from the oven and leave to stand for 10 minutes.

8/ Meanwhile, place the tomatoes and cucumber in a salad bowl and dress with some extra-virgin olive oil and balsamic vinegar. Remove the tart from the pan and cut into wedges, and serve with the salad on the side.

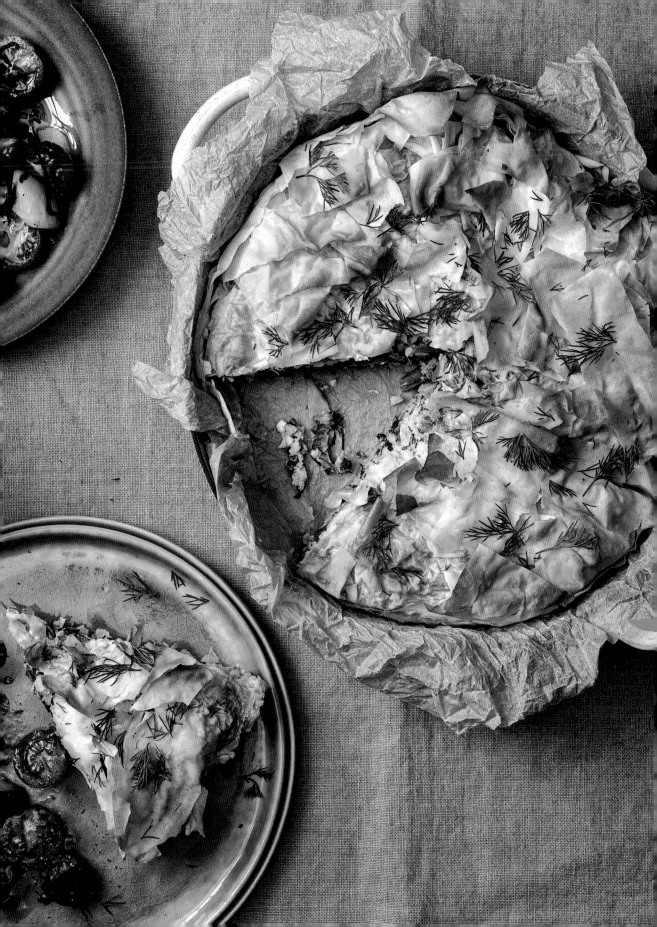

omega-3 salad

Prep time:
5 minutes

Cooking time:
6 minutes

Calories per serving:
581

I know we should never judge on appearances, but this is one good-looking salad. All of the different colours and textures make it perfect to serve at a picnic or on a lunch date. If you don't like mackerel, try this with some smoked salmon or hot salmon fillets, or flake some tinned tuna over the top.

serves 2

2 large free-range eggs

120g long-stem broccoli

100g cos or Little Gem lettuce(s), trimmed and roughly chopped

120g cooked beetroot

6 cherry tomatoes, each cut into little wedges

150g sustainably sourced smoked mackerel fillets, skin removed, broken up

For the dressing

3 tablespoons Greek yoghurt

juice of 1 lemon

2 tablespoons extra-virgin olive oil

sea salt and freshly ground black pepper

1/ Fill a medium-sized saucepan with water and place over a high heat. Bring to the boil, then carefully add the whole eggs. Boil for 6 minutes, adding the broccoli after the first minute (so the broccoli cooks for 5 minutes).

2/ Drain and run the eggs under cold water. Set the broccoli aside.

3/ Divide the lettuce between 2 plates or bowls, then scatter over the beetroot, cherry tomatoes and cooked broccoli.

4/ Take one of the eggs and carefully crack the shell on a hard surface. Roll the egg around so the shell breaks, then peel and rinse with cold water. Repeat with the second egg. Cut the eggs in half then place them on top of the salad. Scatter over the mackerel.

5/ To make the dressing, mix together the yoghurt, lemon juice and oil in a bowl and season with salt and pepper. Drizzle over the whole salad and serve.

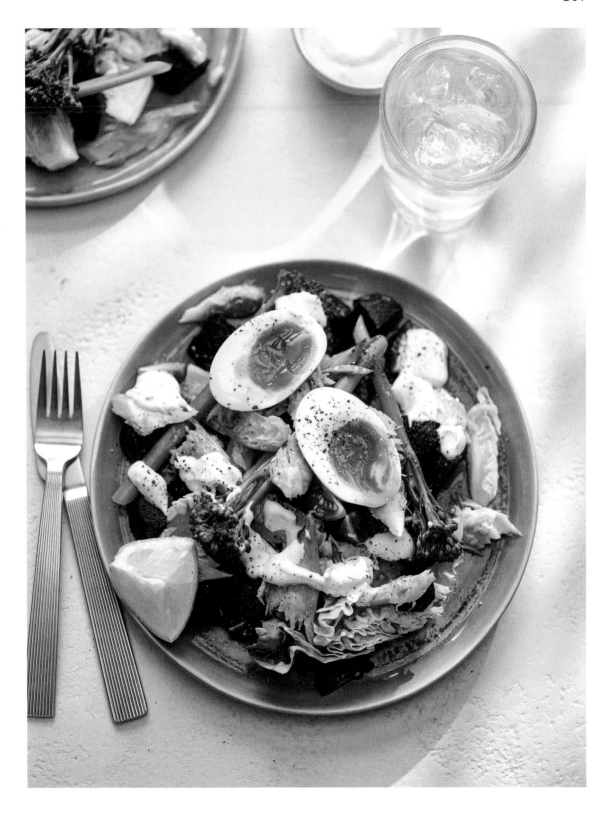

The Ultimate Body Plan for New Mums

green bean & chickpea salad

Prep time:
5 minutes

Cooking time:
3 minutes

Calories per serving:
140

This salad is great on its own – as I'm a veggie, chickpeas are one of my favourite protein sources – but you can also pair it with grilled halloumi, poached salmon or tinned tuna. It's a simple yet delicious way to get lots of fresh ingredients and beans onto one plate.

serves 6

350g green beans, fresh or frozen

1 x 400g tin chickpeas, drained

200g vine tomatoes, roughly chopped

100g cucumber, roughly chopped

½ red chilli, de-seeded and finely sliced

1 tablespoon dried oregano

2 tablespoons red wine vinegar

2 tablespoons extra-virgin olive oil

sea salt and freshly ground black pepper

40g feta cheese, crumbled

1/ Fill a medium-sized saucepan with water and bring to the boil. Add the green beans and cook for 3 minutes until they are cooked but still have a little bite.

2/ Drain the beans and place in a salad bowl. Add the chickpeas, along with the tomatoes and cucumber.

3/ In a small bowl or jug, mix together the chilli, oregano, red wine vinegar and extra-virgin olive oil to make a dressing. Season with salt and pepper, then pour into the salad bowl and give it all a good mix around.

4/ Crumble in the feta and serve.

fridge-raid frittata

Prep time:
5 minutes

Cooking time:
15 minutes

Calories per serving:
279

This is what I make when I have lots of odds and ends left in the fridge or bags of frozen veg to use up. Perfect for getting rid of those half-tins of chickpeas or beans that are always lurking about. Seriously, the idea is in the name: raid your fridge!

serves 4

6 free-range eggs

50g Cheddar, grated, or feta, crumbled

sea salt and freshly ground black pepper

3 tablespoons olive oil

½ small onion, finely chopped

½ red pepper, chopped

80g broccoli, roughly chopped (you can use frozen: just defrost it by placing it in a colander and pouring over some boiling water)

handful of frozen peas, or ½ courgette, grated

4–6 cherry vine tomatoes, roughly chopped

1 tablespoon balsamic vinegar

200g baby spinach leaves

1 tablespoon pine nuts, toasted

1/ Preheat the oven to 220°C/200°C fan/425°F/gas 7.

2/ Crack the eggs into a large bowl and mix together with most of the cheese. Season with black pepper.

3/ Heat 1 tablespoon of the oil in a 26cm non-stick ovenproof frying pan over a medium heat. Add the onion and red pepper and cook for 5 minutes until starting to soften. Add the broccoli, peas or courgette and tomatoes and stir for a further 5 minutes.

4/ Reduce the heat to low, then pour in the eggs and gently mix with all the veg. Cook for a few minutes, then scatter the remaining cheese on top. Transfer the pan to the oven for 5 minutes until golden and cooked through.

5/ Make a quick dressing by mixing the remaining 2 tablespoons oil with the balsamic vinegar in a salad bowl. Season with salt and pepper and add the spinach and pine nuts, then toss to coat in the dressing.

6/ Carefully remove the frittata from the pan onto a board – you can either carefully jiggle it out or flip it out of the pan. Cut it into wedges and serve alongside the dressed spinach salad.

harissa-baked aubergine with salsa

Prep time:
15 minutes

Cooking time:
35 minutes

Calories per serving:
377

You can serve this with brown rice for a bit of added 'oomph' and to make it more substantial, but otherwise it's perfect as is for a light lunch. The salsa acts as a zingy and fresh foil to the kicky aubergine.

serves 4

2 aubergines, trimmed and chopped into 2–3cm chunks

1 heaped tablespoon harissa paste

3 tablespoons olive oil

1 x 400g tin cannellini beans, drained

50g hazelnuts, toasted and roughly chopped

50g feta cheese

100g Greek yoghurt

1 tablespoon tahini

juice of 1 lemon

sea salt and freshly ground black pepper

For the salsa

½ small red onion, finely sliced

300g ripe tomatoes, roughly chopped

small bunch of coriander, leaves picked and stems roughly chopped

1 tablespoon extra-virgin olive oil

1 tablespoon red wine vinegar

1/ Preheat the oven to 200°C/180°C fan/400°F/gas 6.

2/ Place the aubergine chunks in a roasting tray. Rub with the harissa paste and 2 tablespoons of the oil, then cook in the oven for 35 minutes (giving it all a shake about halfway through) until softened and golden.

3/ Meanwhile, make the salsa. Place the onion in a bowl and add the tomatoes, along with half the coriander leaves and all the stems. Stir in the extra-virgin olive oil and red wine vinegar and season with salt and pepper. Give it all a good mix, then set aside.

4/ In a separate bowl, mix together the cannellini beans and most of the hazelnuts, keeping a few back. Stir in the feta and 1 tablespoon of the oil.

5/ To make the dressing, mix together the yoghurt, tahini and lemon juice in a small bowl and season with salt and pepper.

6/ Divide the aubergines between 4 plates and top each one with a portion of the beans, then the salsa and some dollops of the dressing. Scatter over the remaining coriander leaves and reserved toasted hazelnuts and serve.

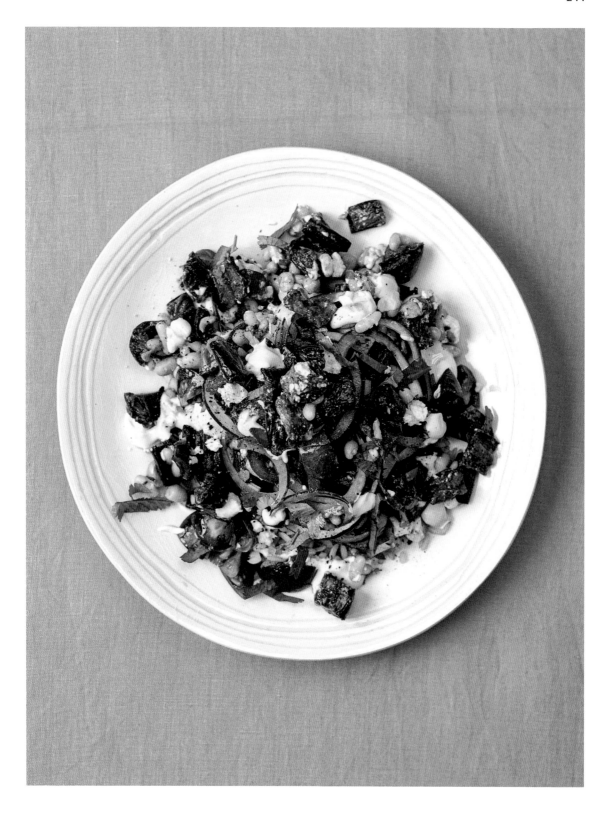

The Ultimate Body Plan for New Mums

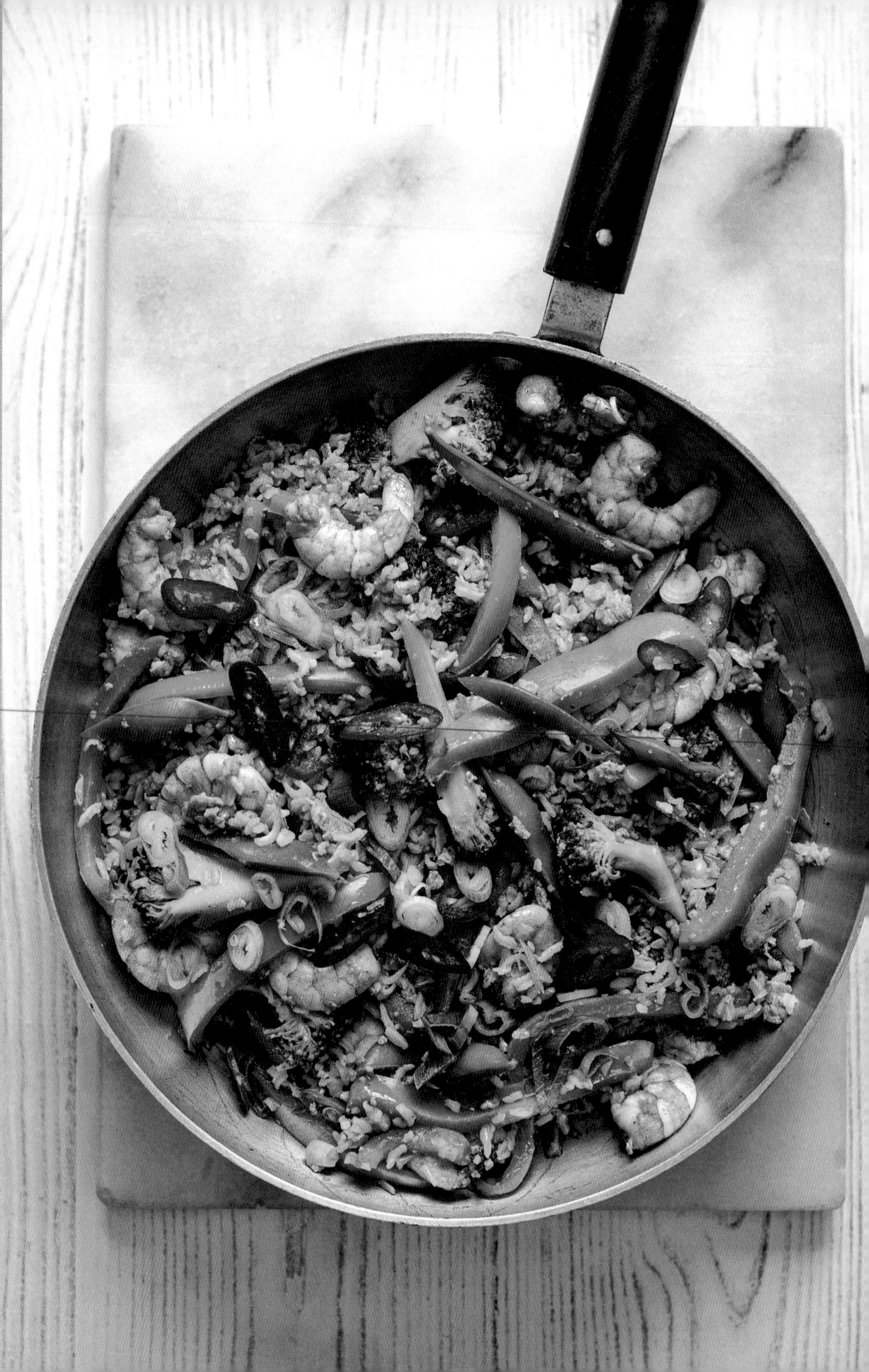

speedy rice & prawns

Prep time:
5 minutes

Cooking time:
15 minutes

Calories per serving:
280

This is one of Gorka's favourite dishes to cook and Mia loves it. It looks fancy but is actually so simple. You just use microwave rice, frozen prawns and a bag of stir-fry veg. Done. (As a veggie, I usually substitute the prawns for tofu.) We always keep a stash of microwave rice in the cupboard, ready for whenever we need an easy lunch or dinner. Any kind will do in this recipe, but brown rice is great for added fibre. Also, feel free to throw in those leftover half peppers that always seem to be in the fridge even though you can't ever remember eating the first half.

serves 4

2 tablespoons olive oil

2 garlic cloves, finely chopped

4 spring onions, trimmed and finely sliced

1 teaspoon mild curry powder

350g mixed bag of stir-fry vegetables (or loose veg cut into bite-sized pieces – try things like peppers, long-stem broccoli, courgette, baby corn and sugar snap peas)

225g frozen king prawns

2 large free-range eggs

1 tablespoon reduced-salt soy sauce

1 x 250g pouch brown basmati microwave rice

1/ Heat the oil in a large wok or frying pan over a medium heat. Add the garlic, spring onions, curry powder and vegetables and cook for 4 minutes, then add the prawns and cook for a further 4 minutes.

2/ Crack the eggs into the pan and add the soy sauce, then mix well to combine. Microwave the rice according to the packet instructions, then add that to the pan, too. Stir to combine, then serve.

super-quick tofu noodles

Prep time:
5 minutes

Cooking time:
10 minutes

Calories per serving:
274

This is what I call a really 'clean' broth: simple flavours, very healthy, and incredibly easy and quick to make. I highly recommend using bouillon veg stock powder if you can find it, as it lasts for ages and can be used for seasoning in soups and stocks.

serves 4

1 tablespoon oil

2cm piece of fresh root ginger, finely sliced

4 spring onions, trimmed and finely sliced

150g greens, such as pak choi, frozen broccoli and/or green beans

150g chestnut mushrooms, sliced

1 red pepper, cut into strips

1¾ pints vegetable stock

280g firm tofu (smoked or normal) cut into 2cm cubes

½ teaspoon demerara or caster sugar

1 tablespoon reduced-salt soy sauce

300g thick udon noodles (choose the quick-cook ones, as they only take 2 minutes!)

1/ Heat the oil in a medium-sized saucepan over a medium heat. Add the ginger, spring onions and your chosen greens, along with the mushrooms, red pepper, vegetable stock, tofu, sugar and soy sauce. Bring to the boil and simmer for 5 minutes, or until the veg is cooked through.

2/ Add the noodles and cook for a further 2 minutes. To serve, divide the noodles between 4 bowls, then add the greens and tofu, and finally pour over the broth.

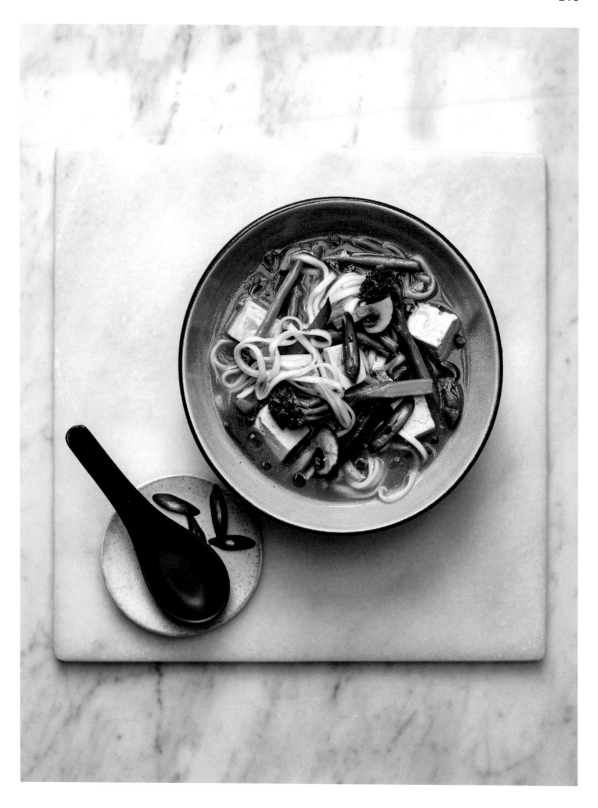

The Ultimate Body Plan for New Mums

cauliflower carbonara

Prep time:
5 minutes

Cooking time:
50 minutes

Calories per serving:
404

A perfect creamy carbonara without using egg or cream (a proper carbonara should never use cream, FYI). To make the recipe vegan, use vegan Parmesan.

serves 4

400g fresh cauliflower, trimmed and cut into bite-sized pieces (stalk and all!), or frozen cauliflower florets

1 tablespoon olive oil

1 tablespoon cumin seeds

sea salt and freshly ground black pepper

1 x 400g tin chickpeas, drained

300g spaghetti

100ml unsweetened fortified oat/almond milk

15g Parmesan (or a veggie/vegan alternative)

handful of rocket, to serve (optional)

1/ Preheat the oven to 200°C/180°C fan/400°F/gas 6.

2/ Place the cauliflower in a roasting tray and drizzle over the olive oil. Scatter over the cumin seeds, some salt and pepper and a good splash of water, then give it all a good shake to coat.

3/ Cover the tray with tin foil and roast for 35 minutes, then remove the foil and add the chickpeas. Continue to cook, uncovered, for a further 15 minutes.

4/ Meanwhile, bring a large saucepan of salted water to the boil and cook the pasta according to the packet instructions, reserving a good mugful of the starchy water before draining.

5/ When the cauliflower and chickpeas are ready, transfer about a third of the contents of the roasting tray to a food-processor. Add the oat or almond milk and blitz to create a creamy paste.

6/ Stir the paste and the rest of the roasted cauliflower and chickpeas into the spaghetti, adding a good splash of the pasta water to create a creamy sauce that coats the pasta.

7/ Serve topped with the Parmesan and rocket (if using.)

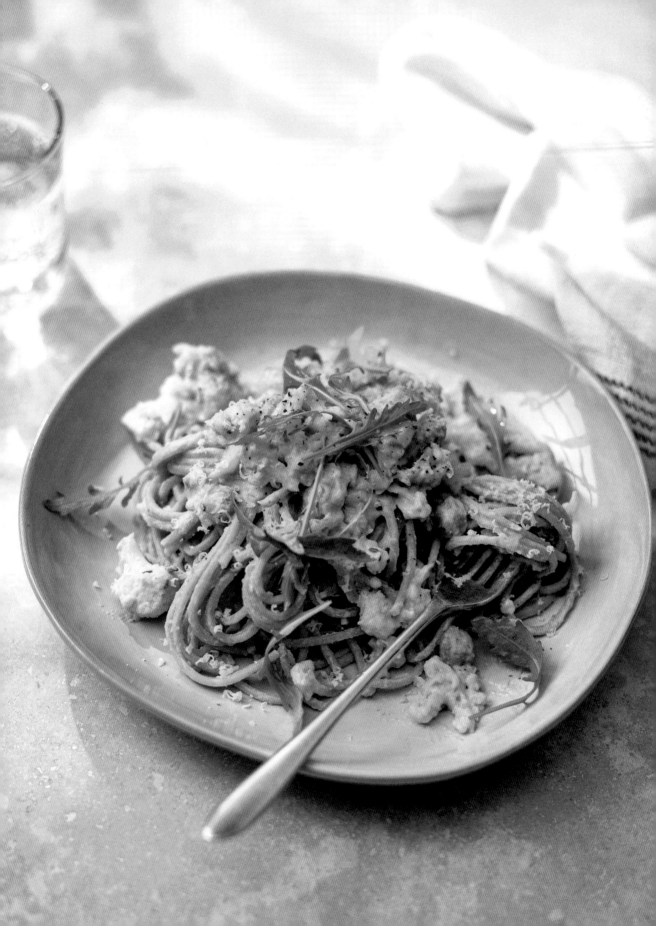

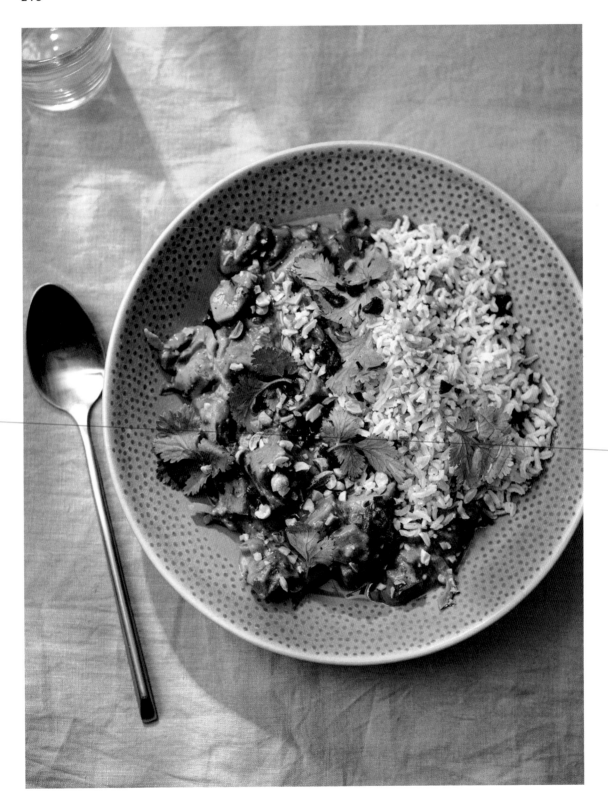

west african stew

Prep time:
5 minutes

Cooking time:
35–45 minutes

Calories per serving:
456

A guest made this on the cooking show I was co-hosting, *Steph's Packed Lunch* on Channel 4, and it was so tasty I decided to create my own veggie version. You can add chicken, fish or prawns if you like. If you can get hold of it, I recommend using frozen okra, but if you can't, courgette will do just fine.

serves 6

1 tablespoon olive oil

1 onion, finely sliced

2 garlic cloves, crushed

1 teaspoon dried chilli flakes

1 teaspoon ground cumin

1 teaspoon ground ginger

handful of coriander, leaves picked and stalks finely chopped

1 red chilli, finely chopped (de-seeded if you don't like it too hot!)

2 sweet potatoes (approx. 500g total), peeled and cut into 2cm chunks

175g fresh or frozen okra, chopped into 1cm pieces, or 1 courgette, halved lengthways then cut into 2cm chunks

1 x 400ml tin light coconut milk

1 x 400g tin plum tomatoes

1 tablespoon tomato purée

500ml vegetable stock

3 tablespoons smooth peanut butter

To serve:
300g steamed rice

30g peanuts, toasted and crushed

1/ Heat the oil in a medium-sized non-stick saucepan over a medium heat. Add the onion, garlic, chilli flakes, cumin and ground ginger, along with the coriander stalks and most of the fresh chilli. Cook for 5–10 minutes, stirring, until the onion starts to soften.

2/ Add the sweet potatoes and okra or courgette and cook for a couple of minutes, then stir in the coconut milk, tinned tomatoes, tomato purée, stock and peanut butter.

3/ Bring to the boil, then reduce the heat to low and simmer for 25–30 minutes until the sweet potatoes are cooked through and the sauce looks thick and yummy.

4/ Serve with steamed rice, and scatter over the coriander leaves, crushed peanuts and the remaining red chilli.

aubergine & sweet potato korma

Prep time:
5 minutes

Cooking time:
25 minutes

Calories per serving:
447

The chicken korma in my first book was such a success that I decided we needed a veggie version. Using your own spices really does make the flavour so much stronger, but a couple of tablespoons of good-quality shop-bought korma paste (not sauce) will work, too – just skip the dried spices and add the paste at the same time as the aubergine.

serves 4

1 tablespoon olive oil

1 red onion, roughly chopped

handful of coriander, leaves picked and stalks finely chopped

2cm piece of fresh root ginger, grated or finely chopped

2 garlic cloves, grated or finely chopped

2 teaspoons cumin seeds

2 teaspoons ground coriander

2 teaspoons garam masala

1 teaspoons ground turmeric

2 aubergines, chopped into 2cm chunks

1 sweet potato, chopped

1 x 400ml tin light coconut milk

1 x 400g tin chickpeas

2 x 250g pouches brown basmati microwave rice

2 tablespoons desiccated coconut

100g fresh or frozen spinach

sea salt and freshly ground black pepper

4 tablespoons Greek yoghurt

lime wedges, to serve

1/ Heat the oil in a large non-stick saucepan over a medium heat. Add the red onion, coriander stalks, ginger, garlic and spices. Cook for 2 minutes, then add the aubergine and keep cooking for a further 8 minutes until the onion has softened and the spices are smelling delicious.

2/ Add the sweet potato, coconut milk and chickpeas (along with their liquid) and cook for 10 minutes, covered, until the sweet potato is cooked through.

3/ Meanwhile, prepare the microwave rice according to the packet instructions.

4/ Stir the desiccated coconut and spinach into the pan and season to taste, adding a little splash of water if needed.

5/ Serve the curry with the basmati rice and a dollop of Greek yoghurt, with the coriander leaves scattered over and lime wedges on the side, for squeezing.

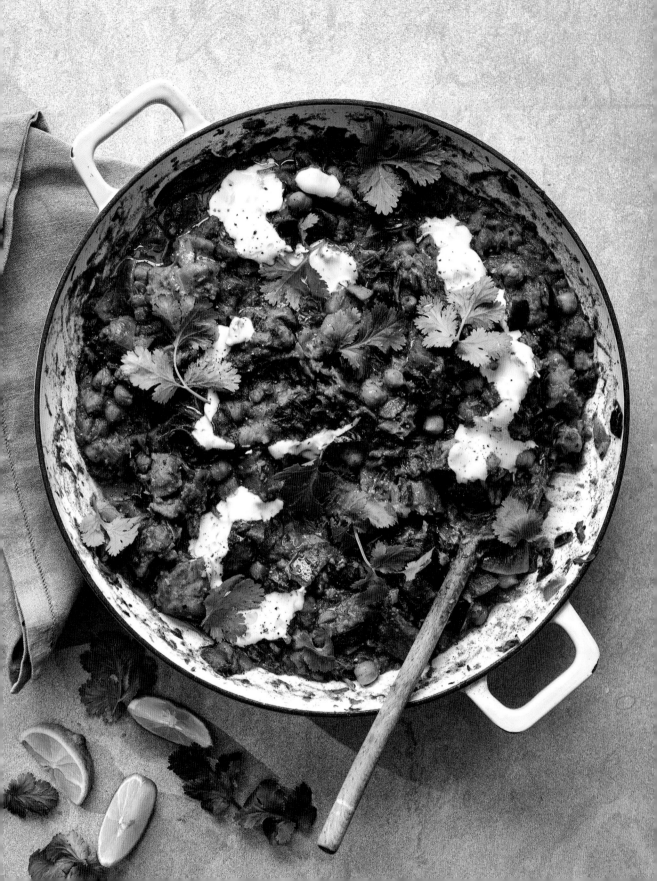

creamy red thai coconut prawn curry

Prep time:
10 minutes

Cooking time:
15 minutes

Calories per serving:
351

Brace yourselves, as this has quite a kick to it. You can use shop-bought paste for this one – and I recommend stocking up on a few jars, as you'll be keen to experiment after trying this. All you have to do is add some veg and frozen prawns (or tofu) and ta-da! A beautiful curry dish in 15 minutes. (Remember to buy paste and not a ready-made sauce. Some brands come in tubs or resealable pouches and last for ages as you only need a little).

serves 4

1 tablespoon vegetable oil

1 onion, sliced

1 garlic clove, finely sliced

1 orange pepper, cut into strips

1 heaped tablespoon good-quality Thai red curry paste

180g frozen large king prawns

1 x 400ml tin light coconut milk

200g baby corn and mangetout, cut into bite-sized pieces

2 x 250g pouches basmati coconut microwave rice

To serve
coriander leaves (optional)

lime wedges

1/ Heat the oil in a non-stick wok or frying pan over a high heat. Add the onion, garlic and pepper and cook, stirring, for 5 minutes, then add the curry paste and prawns and stir. It should all be sizzling nicely.

2/ Pour in the coconut milk, then add the baby corn and mangetout. Stir well and reduce the heat to medium. Cook for 8 minutes until the prawns are cooked through and the sauce has slightly thickened.

3/ Meanwhile, prepare the rice according to the packet instructions.

4/ Serve the curry with the rice, scatter over some coriander (if using), and pop some lime wedges on the side for some extra flavour.

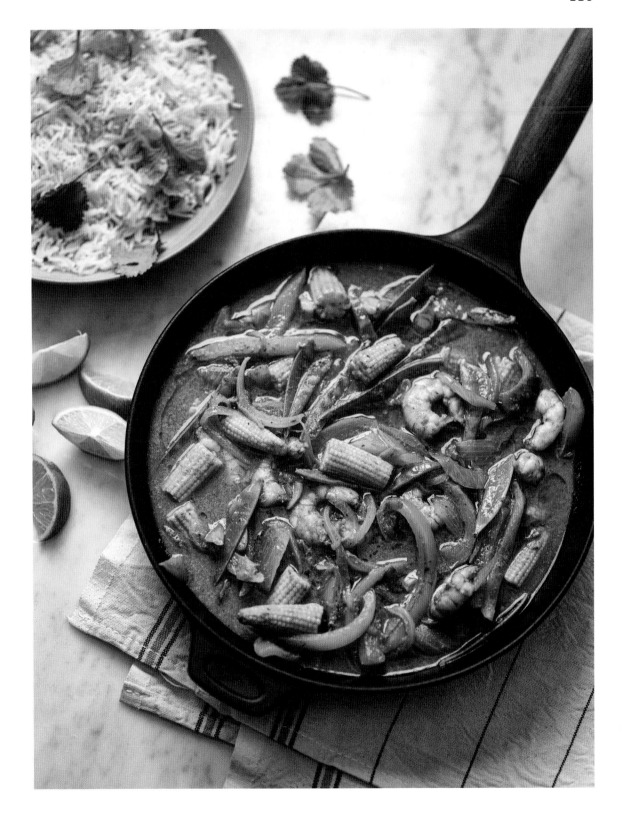

The Ultimate Body Plan for New Mums

creamy chickpea & almond pesto pasta

Prep time:
5 minutes

Cooking time:
10 minutes

Calories per serving:
582

Home-made pesto is one of the great joys of life – and making it earns you major adult points, as only true grown-ups would ever bother. This recipe makes a big batch of the stuff – you only use 6–8 tablespoons of it here – so you can keep the rest in the fridge for another time (it will keep for 2–3 days in a sterilised jar) or even freeze it. Turns out, pesto freezes pretty well. Who knew, eh? My tip is to freeze it in an ice cube tray and then, once frozen, transfer the cubes to a freezer bag, so you can grab a couple whenever needed.

serves 4

50g mixed nuts, such as almonds, hazelnuts or pine nuts

50g Parmesan (or a veggie/vegan alternative), plus extra to serve

1 x 215g tin chickpeas, drained

zest and juice of 1 lemon

50ml extra-virgin olive oil

bunch of basil, leaves picked

300g rigatoni pasta (or another shape, if you prefer!)

1/ Place the nuts and Parmesan in a food-processor and blitz until combined.

2/ Add the chickpeas to the food-processor, along with a good splash of water, the lemon zest and juice, the olive oil and most of the basil (saving some of the smallest leaves for garnish). Blitz again, adding another little splash of water if necessary, to form a pesto.

3/ Cook the pasta in a large saucepan of boiling water according to the packet instructions. Just before you drain the pasta, reserve a mugful of the cooking water and set aside. Drain the pasta as normal, then return it to the pan.

4/ Give the pesto a stir, then add a little of the pasta water to loosen the mix, stirring again until you get the right texture – you want it to be nice and creamy. Stir 6–8 tablespoons of the pesto into the pasta, then serve with a little extra Parmesan and the reserved basil leaves scattered over the top. Perfect!

fennel & courgette spaghetti

Prep time:
5 minutes

Cooking time:
15 minutes

Calories per serving:
318

The aniseed flavour of the fennel here is lovely and subtle when paired with the courgette. This is a really light recipe with hardly any ingredients, so it's perfect to throw together when you know baby-related chaos could recommence at any minute.

serves 4

1 tablespoon olive oil

2 garlic cloves, roughly chopped

1 fennel bulb, trimmed, halved and cut into 1cm slices

2 courgettes, grated

100ml water

zest and juice of 1 lemon

300g wholemeal spaghetti

30g Parmesan or a veggie/vegan alternative, grated

sea salt and freshly ground black pepper

1/ Heat the oil in a medium-sized non-stick saucepan over a medium heat. Add the garlic, fennel and courgettes, and cook for 10 minutes, stirring occasionally so it doesn't stick. Add the water and the lemon juice, then cook for a further 5 minutes.

2/ Meanwhile, bring a large saucepan of salted water to the boil and cook the spaghetti according to the packet instructions, reserving a good mugful of the starchy water before draining.

3/ Stir the drained spaghetti into the pan of cooked fennel and courgette. Add a splash of the reserved pasta water and stir in most of the Parmesan, creating a creamy kind of sauce.

4/ Taste and season, then serve topped with a scattering of lemon zest and the remaining Parmesan.

chicken & aubergine tagine

Prep time:
10 minutes

Cooking time:
1 hour 45 minutes

Calories per serving:
594

A great one to cook in advance (either in the morning or even a day ahead), this Moroccan-inspired dish is the definition of comfort food. You can use a medium-sized butternut squash instead of chicken if you want to keep it veggie. There's no need to peel it – just remove the seeds and chop the flesh into 1cm chunks).

serves 6

1 tablespoon olive oil

1 red onion, roughly chopped

2 carrots, chopped into 2cm pieces

1 large aubergine, cut into chunks

1 teaspoon ground cinnamon

1 teaspoon ground cumin

1 teaspoon ground coriander

small bunch of fresh coriander, leaves picked and stalks finely chopped

700g boneless, skinless free-range chicken thighs

100g dried apricots

2 x 400g tins plum tomatoes

1 x 400g tin chickpeas, drained

1½ pints vegetable stock

sea salt and freshly ground black pepper

To serve

natural yoghurt

prepared couscous

pomegranate seeds

mint leaves

1/ Preheat the oven to 200°C/180°C fan/400°F/gas 6.

2/ Heat the oil in a large ovenproof casserole pan (or tagine, if you have one) over a medium heat.

3/ Add the onion, carrots and aubergine, along with the spices and coriander stalks. Cook for 5 minutes, stirring occasionally so it doesn't stick.

4/ Add the chicken thighs and apricots and cook for a further 5 minutes until the chicken has some colour, then add the tinned tomatoes, chickpeas and stock.

5/ Season well and bring to the boil. Scrunch a large piece of baking paper under running water, then gently place it over the stew. Cover with the lid, then transfer to the oven for 1 hour.

6/ Remove the lid and stir, then cook, uncovered, for a further 30 minutes until the chicken is cooked through and the sauce has thickened. Taste and adjust seasoning if needed.

7/ To serve, dollop a few spoonfuls of natural yoghurt onto the tagine and scatter over the coriander leaves. Jazz up a hot couscous side dish by stirring through some pomegranate seeds and mint. Next, eat as much as you can.

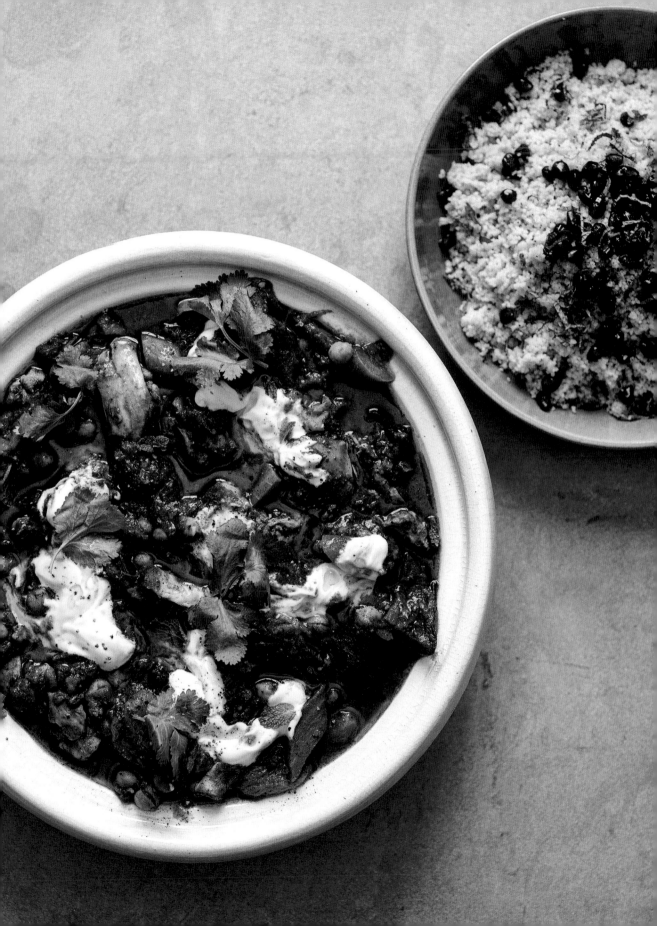

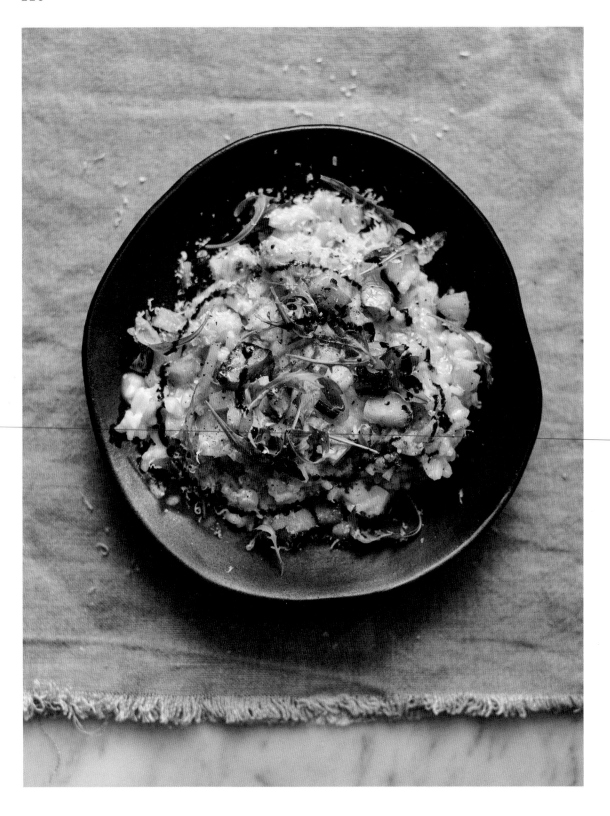

parsnip risotto

Prep time:
10 minutes

Cooking time:
45–50 minutes

Calories per serving:
478

The humble parsnip is a totally underrated vegetable (just roast some with honey and thyme if you don't believe me). This recipe takes a bit of effort, but you can split the method into sections: you can roast the parsnip first and then set it aside for later; and you can prep the risotto base separately (up to the point of adding the parsnips) and leave it to cool until you're ready to put everything together. It's perfect served with rocket and a little balsamic glaze.

serves 4

450g parsnips, peeled and chopped into 2cm pieces

2 tablespoons olive oil

sea salt and freshly ground black pepper

small bunch of thyme, leaves picked

1 tablespoon runny honey

2 celery sticks, finely chopped (as fine as you can!)

1 onion, finely chopped

260g risotto rice

good splash of white wine (or apple juice, if you prefer – but don't worry, the alcohol will burn off anyway)

2½ pints vegetable stock

30g Parmesan, finely grated

rocket dressed with balsamic glaze, to serve

1/ Preheat the oven to 210°C/190°C fan/410°F/gas 6½.

2/ Place the parsnips in a roasting tray and drizzle with 1 tablespoon of the olive oil and a splash of water. Season with salt and pepper and scatter over the thyme leaves. Roast for 35 minutes until golden, then drizzle with the honey and set aside.

3/ Meanwhile, heat the remaining 1 tablespoon oil in a large non-stick sauté pan over a medium heat. Add the celery and onion and cook for 5 minutes until softened. Add the rice and cook for another couple of minutes, then add a splash of white wine (or apple juice). Let the liquid evaporate, then add a ladleful of hot stock. Cook, stirring, until the liquid has been absorbed, then add some more. Keep doing this, adding the stock a ladleful at a time, for 25–30 minutes. During the last 5 minutes of cooking, add three quarters of the roasted parsnips.

4/ When the risotto is ready, the rice grains should be soft but still have a slight bite (al dente). Once you reach this stage, add most of the Parmesan, then pop a lid on the pan and turn off the heat. Leave for 5 minutes.

5/ Serve the risotto with the remaining roasted parsnips, and some balsamic-dressed rocket on the side.

one-tray chicken roast

Prep time:
30 minutes

Cooking time:
1 hour

Calories per serving:
583

This is my take on a quick roast chicken. Using thighs and legs speeds up the cooking process, and the lovely juices soak into the veg in the pan, helping to make a fabulously rich gravy. Don't worry if you don't like Marmite (yeast extract) – it's just to add depth to the flavour. Your gravy won't actually taste of Marmite – I wouldn't put you through that. Of course you can just use shop-bought gravy, but I swear after you've tried your own, you won't go back. (Also, shop-bought gravy powders tend to contain quite a lot of additives, while yours will contain only good things.)

serves 4

8 free-range chicken drumsticks or thighs (or a mix of both)

6 carrots, chopped into 2cm chunks on the diagonal

2 celery sticks, roughly chopped

1 large onion, cut into wedges

1 garlic bulb, halved through the middle of the cloves

750g new potatoes

small bunch of rosemary, leaves picked

2 tablespoons olive oil

sea salt and freshly ground black pepper

2 heaped tablespoons plain flour

1 teaspoon reduced-salt yeast extract (e.g. Marmite)

500ml chicken stock

350g long-stem broccoli, trimmed

1/ Preheat the oven to 220°C/200°C fan/425°F/gas 7.

2/ Place the chicken, carrots, celery, onion, garlic, potatoes and rosemary in a large roasting tray. Drizzle with the olive oil, season with salt and pepper and give it all a good mix about.

3/ Roast for 40–45 minutes, shuffling things about halfway through to make sure everything is getting nice and golden.

4/ To make a quick gravy, remove the onion, celery and half of the carrots and place in a saucepan. Tip up the tray to pour the juices from the chicken into the saucepan. Cover the chicken and remaining veg and set aside to rest, then place the saucepan over a medium heat and mash it all down. Add the flour and stir to create a thick paste, then add the yeast extract and stock. Bring to the boil and cook for 5 minutes, then push the mix through a thick sieve into a clean saucepan. Place over a low heat and simmer to reduce to your desired thickness. (If you prefer, you can just use a ready-made gravy!)

5/ Meanwhile, cook the broccoli in a saucepan of boiling water for 5 minutes until just tender, then drain and serve alongside everything else.

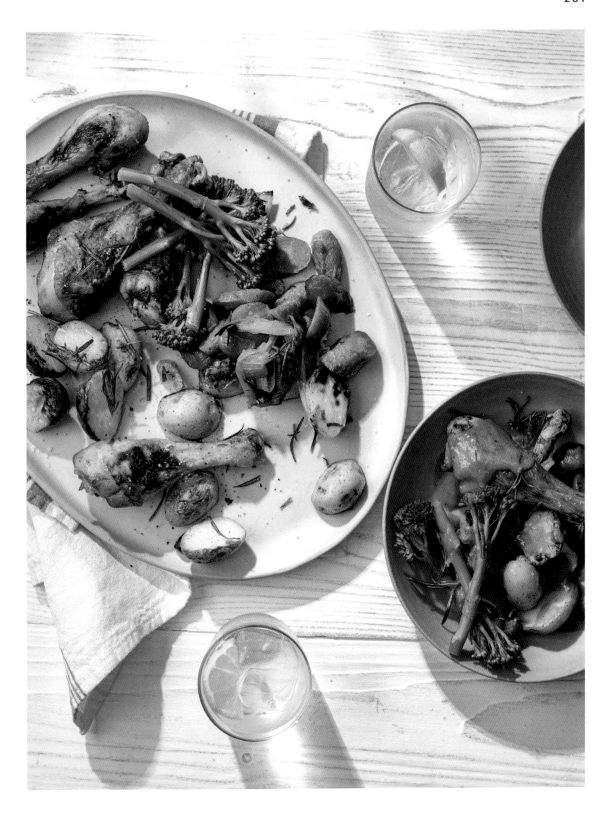

The Ultimate Body Plan for New Mums

one-pot veggie sausage stew

Prep time:
10 minutes

Cooking time:
35–40 minutes

Calories per serving:
338

Right, I'm not on a vegetarian crusade, I swear, but before any meat-eaters dismiss the thought of using veggie sausages in this stew, can I ask you to please just give it a go? I think you'll be really surprised by the quality and taste of what's available nowadays (and veggie versions tend to be healthier, too). This stew is rich, hearty and filling – perfect for cosy nights in front of the TV or for a dinner party with lots of hungry guests.

serves 4

2 tablespoons olive oil

small bunch of rosemary, leaves picked and roughly chopped

2 celery sticks, roughly chopped

1 red onion, cut into wedges

1 red pepper, cut into 8 pieces

pinch of dried chilli flakes

1 teaspoon smoked paprika

10 meat-free chipolatas (or higher-welfare pork chipolata sausages)

150ml red wine

2 x 400g tins plum tomatoes

500g new potatoes (or large waxy potatoes, cut into bite-sized pieces)

1 x 400g tin cannellini beans (or other white beans or chickpeas), drained

100g kale, stalks removed, torn into bite-sized pieces

1/ Heat the olive oil in a large casserole pan over a medium heat. Add the rosemary, celery, onion and pepper. Stir in the chilli flakes and smoked paprika and cook for 5 minutes, or until the vegetables are starting to soften and colour a little.

2/ Add the chipolatas and cook for 3–5 minutes until it is all smelling lovely and the chipolatas are getting nice and golden.

3/ Pour in the red wine and let it cook off a little – just a few minutes will do – then add the tomatoes, potatoes and cannellini beans. Refill one of the tomato tins with water and add that, too. Bring to the boil, then reduce the heat to low, cover with the lid and simmer for 20 minutes.

4/ Remove the lid from the pan, add the kale and cook for a final 5 minutes. Eat while cuddled up watching the latest Scandi detective boxset.

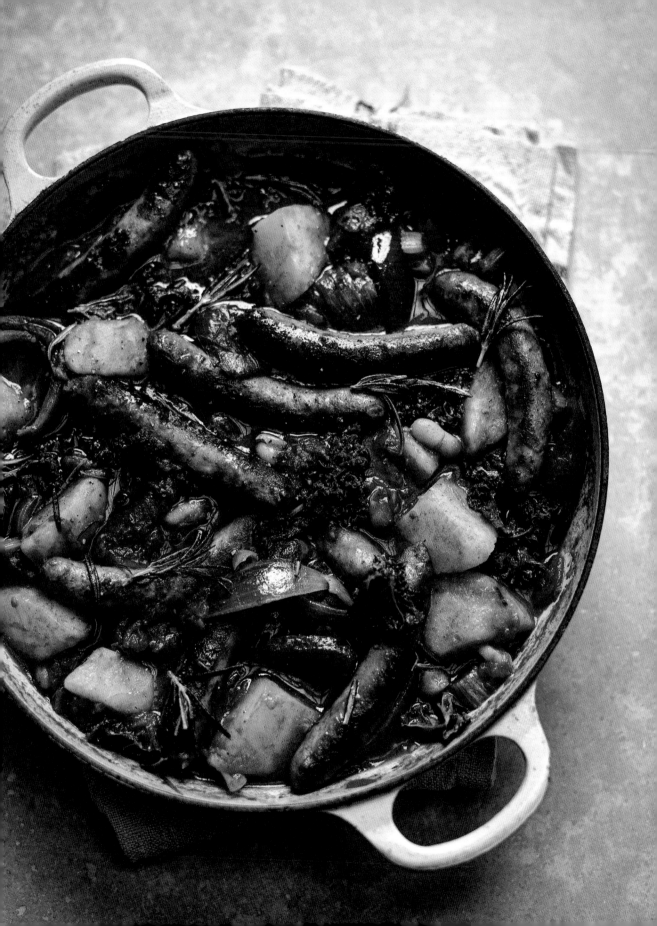

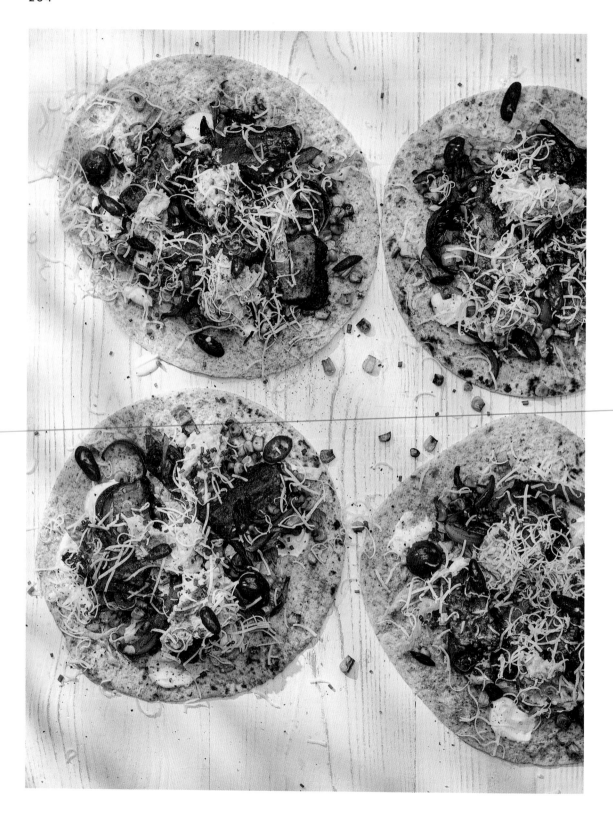

'tex-mex' steak fajitas

Prep time:
5 minutes

Cooking time:
12–14 minutes

Calories per serving:
445

This is a clever way of making a bit of steak go a long way. Make sure to cook this dish over a really high heat for that lovely charred flavour (and smell) reminiscent of summer barbecues.

serves 6

320g sirloin steak

2 tablespoons olive oil

sachet of fajita mix (or, to make your own, mix together 1 teaspoon smoked paprika, 1 teaspoon ground cumin and 1 teaspoon mild chilli powder)

sea salt and freshly ground black pepper

200g tinned sweetcorn, drained

1 orange or red pepper, cut into strips

1 red onion, cut into wedges

handful of ripe cherry tomatoes

To serve

6 wholemeal tortilla wraps, lightly toasted

2 handfuls of shredded lettuce

2 avocados, peeled, stoned and mashed

150ml soured cream

30g Cheddar, grated

small bunch of chives, finely chopped

red chilli slices (optional)

1/ Place a large frying pan over a high heat. Place the steak on a chopping board and drizzle with 1 tablespoon of the olive oil, then rub with the spice mix. Season with salt and pepper.

2/ Place the steak in the hot pan and cook for 2–3 minutes on each side. Once cooked, transfer to a plate and leave to rest.

3/ Keeping the pan on the heat, add the remaining 1 tablespoon oil. Add the sweetcorn, pepper and onion and cook for 6 minutes, stirring every few minutes – it should be sizzling and smelling lovely.

4/ Add the tomatoes and cook for a further 2 minutes, then turn off the heat. Slice the steak into strips and toss it back into the pan, along with any resting juices. Stir to mix everything together.

5/ Serve the steak in the toasted wholemeal tortilla wraps, topped with lettuce, avocado, soured cream, Cheddar, chives and some red chilli (if you like it hot).

teriyaki salmon with garlic greens & rice

Prep time:
5 minutes

Cooking time:
11–15 minutes

Calories per serving:
526

A delicious and filling meal, this Asian-inspired classic is perfect to use up any leftover or frozen greens like spinach, broccoli, peas or kale. (You can add the spinach, peas or kale straight to the pan, but blanch the broccoli first.)

serves 4

2 tablespoons teriyaki sauce

2 tablespoons reduced-salt soy sauce

2 tablespoons sweet chilli sauce

4 sustainably sourced skin-on salmon fillets (approx. 110g each)

250g brown rice (or 2 x 250g pouches brown microwave rice)

400g mixed greens, including long-stem broccoli, green beans and asparagus

2 tablespoons sesame oil

1 heaped tablespoon sesame seeds, toasted

1 garlic clove, finely grated

handful of fresh coriander, leaves picked

lime wedges, to serve (optional)

1/ In a shallow bowl big enough to hold the salmon fillets, mix together the teriyaki sauce, soy sauce and sweet chilli sauce. Add the salmon fillets (skin-side up) and leave to marinate. Set aside whilst you prep the other bits.

2/ Cook the rice according to the packet instructions. (If you're using microwave rice, you can do this just before serving.)

3/ Meanwhile, place a medium-sized non-stick frying pan over a high heat. Add the salmon and cook for 8–10 minutes, turning halfway, until it's cooked through and the skin is lovely and crispy. Add any remaining marinade to the pan for the last few minutes to coat the salmon and give it a nice dark colour.

4/ Fill a medium-sized saucepan with water and bring to the boil. Add the greens and cook for 3–5 minutes, then drain.

5/ In a small bowl, mix together the sesame oil, sesame seeds and grated garlic. Pour this mixture over the hot greens.

6/ If you're using microwave rice, prepare it now. Serve the salmon and greens on a bed of rice, drizzling over the extra marinade from the pan. Sprinkle over the coriander leaves and serve, with lime wedges on the side for squeezing.

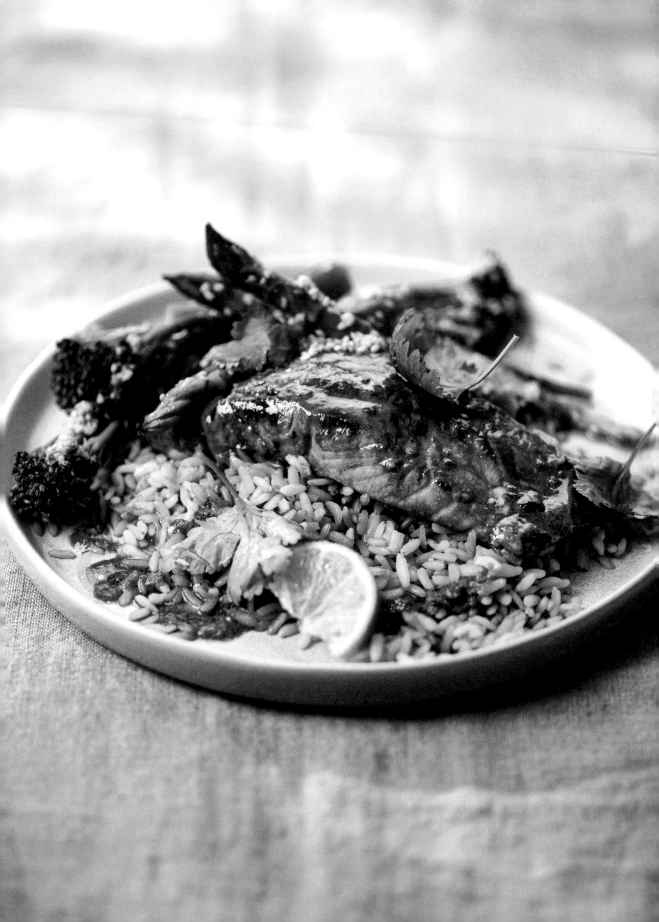

cheesy chicken burger with sweet potato wedges

Prep time:
5 minutes

Cooking time:
30 minutes

Calories per serving:
569

Ahh, a guilt-free burger and chips! Well, kind of. No burger-and-chips dish is totally guilt-free, but this comes pretty close. The chicken and leek patty is accompanied by grated carrot, lettuce and tomato, so the dish is packed with veggies. The sweet potato is baked instead of fried (plus sweet potato counts as one of your five a day – true story) and you can use wholemeal rolls instead of white for added fibre. Result.

serves 6

2 sweet potatoes, cut into wedges

3 tablespoons olive oil

sea salt and freshly ground black pepper

2 leeks, trimmed and roughly chopped

500g free-range chicken thighs, skin and bones removed (prepared weight approx. 430g)

2 garlic cloves, peeled

10g flat-leaf parsley

30g Parmesan

2 teaspoons wholegrain mustard

50g breadcrumbs

6 wholemeal bread rolls or burger buns, halved

2 large vine tomatoes, sliced

2 carrots, grated

2 Little Gem lettuces, leaves separated, or 2 handfuls of salad leaves

tomato ketchup and mayonnaise, to serve (optional)

1/ Preheat the oven to 200°C/180°C fan/400°F/gas 6 and line a baking tray with tin foil. Place the sweet potato wedges on the prepared baking tray and drizzle over 2 tablespoons of the olive oil. Season with salt and pepper and place in the oven for 30 minutes, giving them a good shuffle about halfway through.

2/ Meanwhile, place the leeks in a food-processor and pulse until finely chopped. Add the chicken, garlic, parsley, Parmesan and mustard. Pulse it all again until the chicken is cut up and the mixture forms a kind of paste.

3/ Season well and transfer to a bowl, then use your hands to mould the mixture into 6 round patties. Carefully flatten them to a thickness of around 2cm. Place the breadcrumbs in a shallow dish and dip the patties into them, turning to coat on both sides, then place on a tray or plate lined with baking paper. Cover and leave to rest for 10 minutes in the fridge.

4/ Heat the remaining 1 tablespoon oil in a medium-sized ovenproof frying pan over a medium heat. Remove the patties from the fridge and fry for 5 minutes on each side, until golden and crisp on the surface. Transfer the pan with the patties to the oven to cook for a further 5 minutes.

5/ To assemble, toast the rolls and place a burger in each one, along with a slice of tomato and some carrot and lettuce. Add a little mayo or ketchup (if using) and serve with the sweet potato wedges.

creamy pasta bake

Prep time:
10 minutes

Cooking time:
50–55 minutes

Calories per serving:
597

This is a mix between a pasta bake, a fish pie and a corn chowder – with lots of added veggies. Vegetarians can just leave out the fish and it'll still taste great.

serves 6

500g pasta

3 tablespoons olive oil

1 onion, sliced

2 leeks, trimmed and chopped

small bunch of flat-leaf parsley, stalks finely chopped, leaves roughly chopped

2 heaped tablespoons plain flour

500ml cow's milk or unsweetened fortified oat milk

500ml vegetable stock

70g Cheddar, grated

sea salt and freshly ground black pepper

400g frozen white fish fillets (or smoked haddock, if you can get it)

100g broccoli florets

200g frozen sweetcorn

60g slightly stale wholemeal bread

1 garlic clove, finely chopped

1/ Preheat the oven to 210°C/190°C fan/410°F/gas 6½.

2/ Fill a large saucepan with water and bring to the boil. Add the pasta and cook for 5 minutes, then drain. Return the pasta to the pan and set aside.

3/ Meanwhile, heat 2 tablespoons of the oil in a large non-stick saucepan over a medium heat. Add the onion, leeks and parsley. Cook for 10 minutes, stirring occasionally, then add the flour. Stir for a few minutes until the flour forms a paste, then add a splash of the milk and stir again.

4/ Slowly add the remaining milk, a little at a time, stirring until a nice thick sauce is formed. Add the stock and cheese, season with salt and pepper, and give it all a good stir.

5/ Add the fish, broccoli and sweetcorn and cook for 5 minutes before breaking up the fish a little with the spoon.

6/ Pour the mixture into the pasta pan and mix together, then transfer into a 30 x 20cm ovenproof dish.

7/ Place the bread, garlic and remaining 1 tablespoon olive oil in a mini blender and blitz to create breadcrumbs. Sprinkle on top of the pasta bake.

8/ Cook for 30–35 minutes until crispy and bubbling.

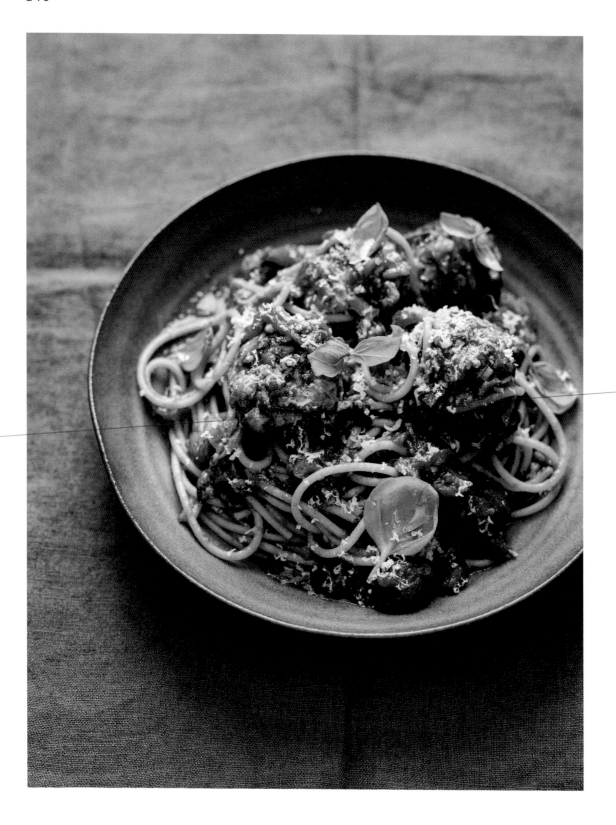

turkey meatballs

Prep time:
20 minutes

Cooking time:
15–20 minutes

Calories per serving:
529

Every good cook should have a solid meatball recipe in their arsenal, and this is mine. Here, I've used turkey, which is lower in fat than the usual beef. I've also hidden some veg within the mince mix – a great way to sneak it past the kids.

serves 6

1 tablespoon fennel seeds

1 small onion, finely chopped

3 garlic cloves, crushed or finely chopped

500g lean turkey mince

150g breadcrumbs

zest of 1 lemon

1 courgette, grated

1 large free-range egg

sea salt and freshly ground black pepper

1 tablespoon olive oil

2 x 400g tins plum tomatoes

bunch of basil, stalks finely chopped and half the leaves left whole, half roughly chopped

400g wholemeal spaghetti

30g Parmesan

1/ Bash the fennel seeds into a powder using a pestle and mortar (or blitz in a blender), then place in a bowl. Add the onion and 1 garlic clove, along with the turkey mince, breadcrumbs and lemon zest. Mix to combine.

2/ Squeeze the grated courgette in handfuls to squish out as much moisture as you can, then add to the bowl, along with the egg. Season well and give it all a good mix, then mould into balls about the size of a golf ball – you should get about 25.

3/ Heat the oil in a large non-stick frying pan over a medium heat. Once the pan is hot, add the meatballs and cook for 3–5 minutes, turning occasionally so they get nice and golden all over.

4/ Push the meatballs to one side of the pan, then add the remaining garlic, along with the tinned tomatoes, basil stalks and chopped leaves. Mix this together and cook for 5–10 minutes until the sauce thickens, then stir into the meatballs.

5/ Meanwhile, bring a large saucepan of salted water to the boil and cook the spaghetti according to the packet instructions, reserving a good mugful of the starchy water before draining.

6/ Mix the spaghetti into the meatballs and sauce, adding a splash of the reserved pasta water and stirring until the sauce is all silky. Taste and season, adding more salt and pepper if needed.

7/ Serve with the reserved basil leaves sprinkled on top, and finish with a little grating of Parmesan.

ratatouille

Prep time:
10 minutes

Cooking time:
1 hour 10 minutes

Calories per serving:
235

Can anyone cook this dish without thinking of a tiny chef-rat? I know I can't. The success here is all down to prep. Once that's done, it's very easy: roast everything off, mix it all together in a large pan, add the tinned tomatoes and leave it in the oven, bubbling away. You can freeze leftover portions to enjoy another time, or to add to other dishes.

serves 6

1 large onion, cut into wedges

1 garlic bulb, halved through the middle of the cloves

1 large aubergine, chopped into 2cm chunks

4 ripe plum tomatoes, halved

2 courgettes, chopped into 2cm chunks

2 yellow peppers, chopped into large chunks

2 tablespoons olive oil

sea salt and freshly ground black pepper

2 teaspoons dried mixed herbs

2 x 400g tins plum tomatoes

handful of basil, leaves picked

cooked brown rice or wholemeal pasta, to serve

1/ Preheat the oven to 200°C/180°C fan/400°F/gas 6.

2/ Place all the vegetables in a large roasting tray (or 2 smaller roasting trays). Drizzle with the oil and season with salt, pepper and mixed herbs.

3/ Roast for 1 hour, or until the vegetables are golden and cooked through.

4/ Squeeze the individual garlic cloves out of their skins and return them to the pan. Add the tinned tomatoes, mashing them into the roasted veg, then return to the oven and cook for a further 10 minutes. Taste and adjust the seasoning, then stir in the basil just before serving.

5/ Serve with steamed rice or wholemeal pasta. This is also delicious served over a jacket potato. You could even chop the veg smaller to make a less chunky texture and serve on mini toasts as a little canapé when your pals come over for a glass of wine (which you'll be able to drink after you've finished the training plan, of course).

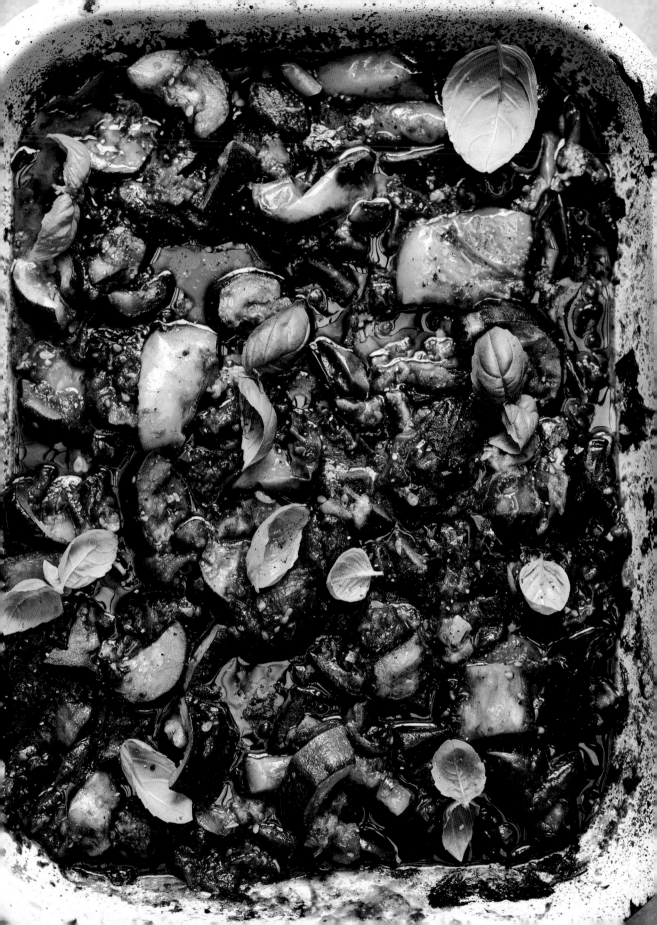

chickpea & mushroom burger

Prep time:
**10 minutes
(plus 30+ minutes
chilling)**

Cooking time:
30 minutes

Calories per serving:
578

Another great burger dish – this time a vegetarian version that will appeal to both veggies and meat-eaters alike. It's fun to use mushrooms in a different way, and chickpeas are super versatile, so it's always handy to have a couple of tins in the cupboard. These burgers store well in the fridge and will keep for 3–5 days, so are good to make ahead of time.

serves 4

2 tablespoons olive oil

200g chestnut mushrooms, sliced

1 teaspoon ground cumin

6 spring onions, trimmed and roughly chopped

150g frozen peas

2 x 400g tins chickpeas, drained

sea salt and freshly ground black pepper

2 tablespoons plain flour

2 tablespoons mixed seeds (sunflower, pumpkin and sesame all work really well)

4 wholemeal burger buns

4 teaspoons tomato ketchup (optional)

4 teaspoons mayonnaise (optional)

2 large vine tomatoes, sliced

¼ cucumber, finely sliced

2 Little Gem lettuces, leaves separated, or a few handfuls of rocket or spinach

1/ Heat 1 tablespoon of the oil in a medium-sized non-stick saucepan over a medium heat. Add the mushrooms, cumin and spring onions and cook for 8 minutes, stirring occasionally. Transfer to a bowl and leave to cool a little.

2/ Place the frozen peas and chickpeas in a food-processor and pulse until the mixture comes together a little. Add the cooked mushroom and spring onion mix and pulse until you have a thick paste that still has some texture. Transfer to a bowl and season generously, then add the flour and seeds and give it a mix.

3/ Using your hands, mould the mix into 4 round patties approx. 10–12cm in diameter and place on a tray lined with baking paper. Cover and chill for at least 30 minutes (preferably 1 hour) to firm up.

4/ Heat the remaining 1 tablespoon of olive oil in a non-stick frying pan over a medium heat and cook the burgers for 5 minutes on each side until crispy and golden brown. Be very careful when you turn them and don't be tempted to turn them too early as this might break the burger – you need to create a crisp little bottom!

5/ Add the burger buns to the pan for the final 5 minutes to toast.

6/ To assemble a burger, spread the bottom of the bun with some tomato ketchup (if using), then top with a burger, followed by mayo (if using), slices of tomato and cucumber, a little lettuce or some salad leaves, and finally the lid.

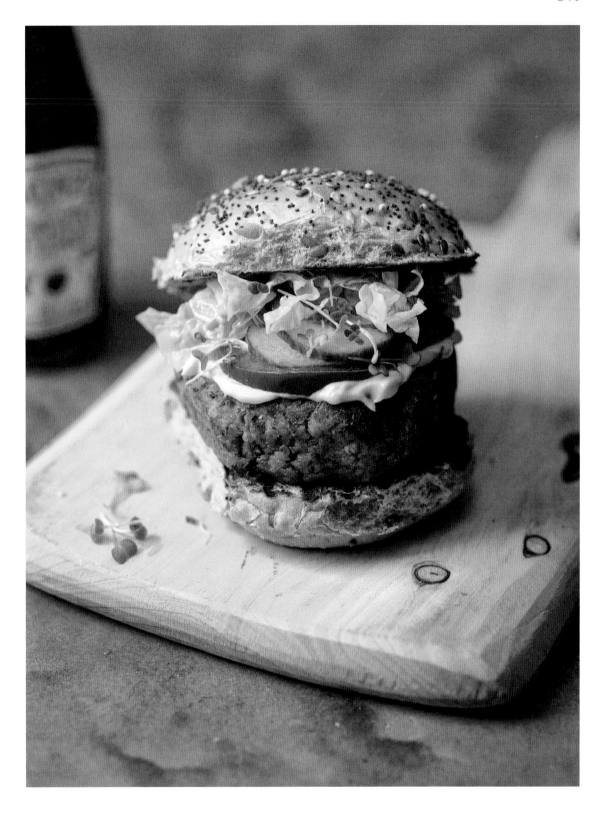

The Ultimate Body Plan for New Mums

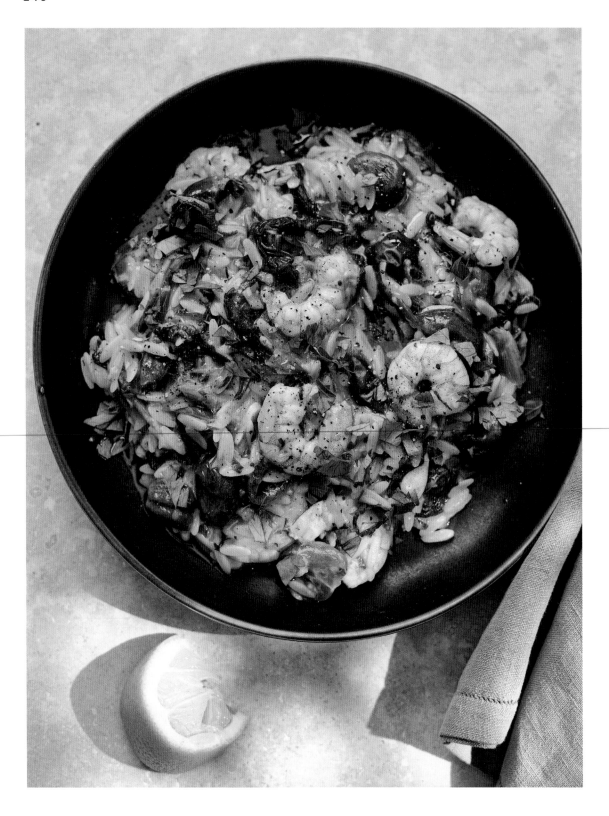

orzo, prawns & greens

Prep time:
5 minutes

Cooking time:
15–20 minutes

Calories per serving:
434

Orzo (also called risoni) is a form of pasta that looks like rice. It's a really easy ingredient to use and works well in salads, risottos and hot dishes like this one. Kids will love this because of the soft, smooth texture and comforting tomato and garlic flavours. You can always throw in more frozen veg if you fancy – peas and broccoli work brilliantly – just make sure that everything is fully cooked through.

serves 4

1 tablespoon olive oil

2 garlic cloves, finely sliced

small bunch of flat-leaf parsley, stalks finely chopped and leaves roughly chopped

1 courgette, grated

500g cherry vine tomatoes, halved

300g orzo

1¼ pints vegetable stock

150g spinach (fresh or frozen)

400g large frozen king prawns

lemon wedges, to serve

1/ Heat the oil in a medium-sized casserole pan over a medium heat. Add the garlic and parsley stalks and cook for a few minutes until the garlic is slightly golden, then add the courgette and tomatoes and keep cooking for 5–8 minutes, stirring occasionally.

2/ Add the orzo, vegetable stock, spinach and prawns and bring to the boil, then cover, reduce the heat to low and simmer for 5 minutes. Remove the lid and simmer for a further 5 minutes, uncovered, until the prawns and orzo are cooked through and the spinach has wilted.

3/ Serve with the parsley leaves scattered on top and lemon wedges, for squeezing.

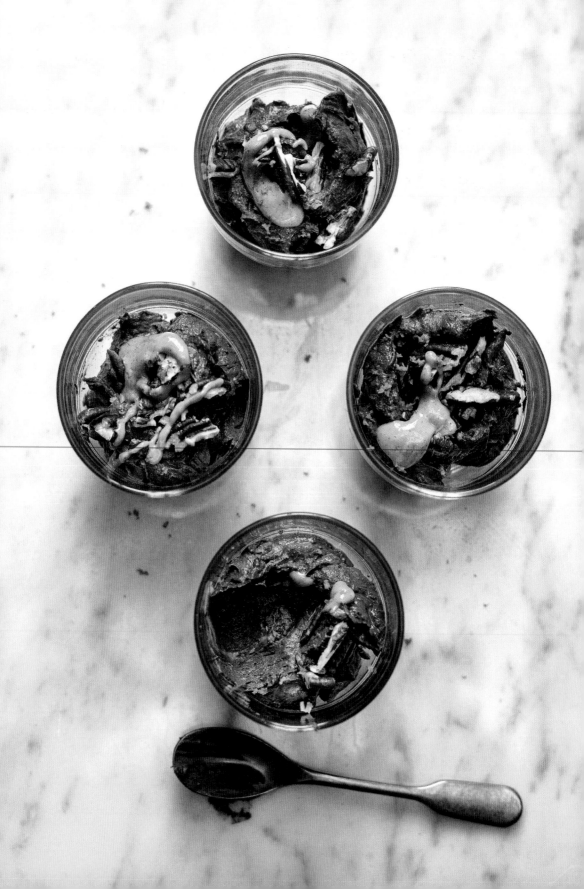

orange choc & nut pots

Prep time:
5 minutes

Cooking time:
3–5 minutes

Calories per serving:
255

These pots can be totally vegan if you use dairy-free chocolate and replace the honey with maple syrup. They're super smooth and satisfying, and you can make them ahead of time if you're having friends over – just keep them covered in a cool place if serving that day. If not, they will keep for 2–3 days in the fridge – just remove 20 minutes before serving.

serves 6

100g dark chocolate (80% cocoa solids), finely chopped

350g silken tofu

60g soft or Medjool dates, stoned

2 teaspoons maple syrup

pinch of ground cinnamon

zest and juice of 1 large orange

2 tablespoons good-quality smooth peanut butter, plus extra to serve

40g pecans, toasted and roughly chopped, to serve

1/ Place a small non-stick saucepan over a medium heat and add the chocolate. Heat for 3–5 minutes, stirring continuously, until melted, then remove from the heat. (If you prefer, you can heat it on medium in a microwave until melted.) Set aside.

2/ Line a bowl with a clean tea towel. Place the tofu in the middle of the tea towel, then gather the edges of the towel together and use it to squeeze out any excess moisture.

3/ Place the squeezed tofu in a food-processor with the dates, maple syrup, cinnamon and orange juice. Blitz until smooth.

4/ Add the melted chocolate and pulse until combined, then transfer the mixture to a bowl.

5/ Add the peanut butter and swirl it into the mixture, then divide between 4 little serving glasses. Top with the toasted nuts, orange zest and a little extra peanut butter.

6/ Eat immediately, or keep covered in a cool place for up to 1 hour before serving.

blueberry & banana loaf

Prep time:
10 minutes

Cooking time:
40–45 minutes

Calories per serving:
276

How many banana loaves do you think were made during lockdown? Hundreds? Thousands? Millions?! I know I made a few (far too many, in fact). This time, we're jazzing things up by adding blueberries (frozen blueberries are fine to use, but will be wetter in texture, so you may need to add an additional tablespoon of flour). Make sure the bananas are properly ripe, otherwise the flavour will be less sweet and the texture less gooey. Also, go with whatever you fancy as far as nuts are concerned: the more, the merrier!

serves 10

2 large, ripe bananas, mashed

4 tablespoons maple syrup

150ml unsweetened fortified oat milk

150g blueberries

100g coconut oil, melted

2 tablespoons smooth peanut butter or Mixed Nut Butter (see page 164)

200g wholemeal self-raising flour

1–2 teaspoons baking powder

60g pecans, almonds or hazelnuts, roughly chopped

1/ Preheat the oven to 200°C/180°C fan/400°F/gas 6 and line a 450g loaf tin with baking paper.

2/ In a large bowl, mix together the mashed bananas, maple syrup, oat milk, blueberries, coconut oil and peanut butter or nut butter. Add the flour, baking powder and nuts and stir until combined.

3/ Pour the mixture into the prepared loaf tin and bake for 40–45 minutes, or until a skewer inserted into the centre comes out clean.

4/ Remove from the oven and leave to cool in the tin for 5 minutes before removing and placing on a cooling rack for a further 15–20 minutes. Eat warm, or enjoy the next day, toasted, with a little extra nut butter spread on top and a cup of tea on the side! The loaf will keep in an airtight container for up to 3 days.

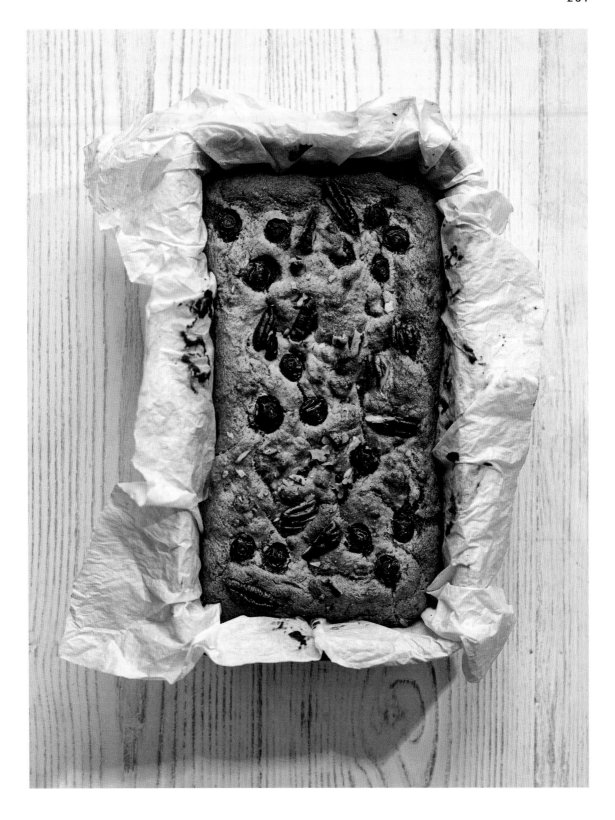

flapjack square bites

Prep time:
10 minutes

Cooking time:
25–30 minutes

Calories per serving:
177

These square bites of deliciousness are perfect to make in bulk. Just store in an airtight container and grab during the week whenever you're in need of an energy boost. They contain lots of seeds, nuts and chia, which are a great source of fibre and protein.

makes 16 flapjacks

4 tablespoons chia seeds

175g rolled oats

100g pistachios, hazelnuts or a mixture of both

4 tablespoons smooth peanut butter or Mixed Nut Butter (see page 164)

4 tablespoons runny honey

3 tablespoons coconut oil

1 pear or apple, grated

50g sultanas

1/ Preheat the oven to 200°C/180°C fan/400°F/gas 6 and line a 20cm square baking tin with baking paper.

2/ Place the chia seeds into a bowl and add 6 tablespoons of warm water. Stir, then set aside. The gel-like substance they will form will help to bind the flapjacks.

3/ Place the oats and nuts in a food-processor and pulse to form an oaty, nutty coarse flour.

4/ Place a small non-stick saucepan over a medium heat and add the peanut butter, honey and coconut oil. Stir until melted and mixed together. Remove from the heat and set aside.

5/ Squeeze the grated apple or pear to remove some of the liquid, then add to the saucepan, along with the chia seed mixture and the sultanas. Give it all a good mix, then pour into the prepared tin, pressing it down so the surface is roughly even. Bake for 25–30 minutes until lightly golden and holding its shape.

6/ Remove from the tin, then cool on a wire rack for 15 minutes before cutting into 16 bite-sized squares. These will keep in an airtight container for up to 1 week but are best eaten within the first few days.

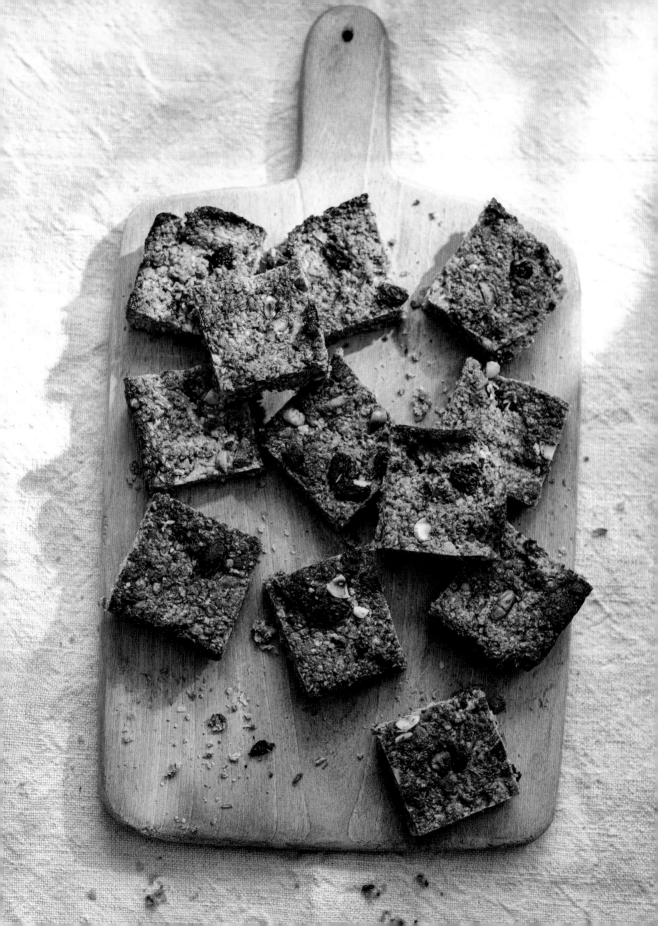

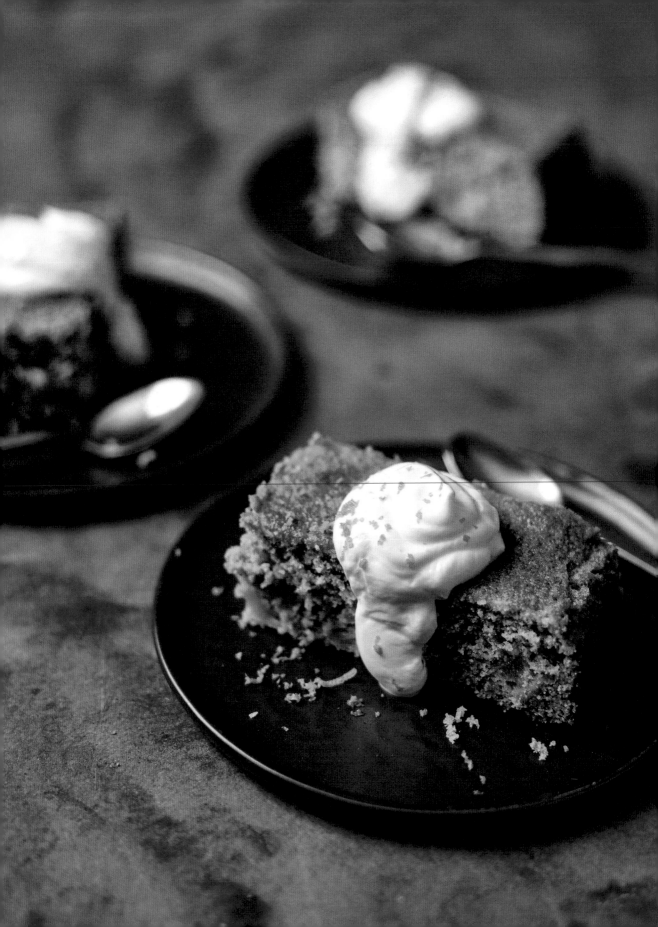

pineapple cake

Prep time:
5 minutes

Cooking time:
25 minutes

Calories per serving:
318

Inspired by a classic upside-down cake, this recipe makes the most of the pineapple by mixing it through instead. I used wholemeal flour here instead of plain, as it adds a nice nutty flavour and is higher in fibre.

serves 8

150g unsalted butter, softened, plus extra for greasing

150ml maple syrup

2 large free-range eggs

1 x 227g tin pineapple slices in juice, roughly chopped and juice reserved

180g wholemeal self-raising flour

1 teaspoon baking powder

150g Greek yoghurt (optional)

1/ Preheat the oven to 200°C/180°C fan/400°F/gas 6 and grease and line a 20cm round cake tin with baking paper.

2/ In a large bowl, mix together the butter and maple syrup. Add the eggs, pineapple and pineapple juice and mix to combine. Sift in the flour and baking powder and mix again, then transfer the mixture to the lined tin.

3/ Bake for 25 minutes, or until a skewer inserted into the centre comes out clean. Cool in the tin for 5 minutes, then transfer to a wire rack to cool for a further 10–15 minutes before slicing.

4/ Serve just as it is, or with a dollop of Greek yoghurt (or custard!). The cake will keep for 3–4 days in an airtight container.

beetroot & chocolate cupcakes

Prep time:
5 minutes

Cooking time:
20 minutes

Calories per cupcake:
195 (based on 16 cupcakes)

Beetroot and chocolate is another one of those mad flavour combinations that, for some reason, just absolutely works. I've used dates for their intense caramelly flavour, and wholemeal flour for a nutty edge. You can also use this recipe to make one big cake. Just put the mixture into a greased cake tin instead of cupcake moulds and bake for 30–40 minutes, or until your testing skewer comes out clean.

makes 16–18 cupcakes

100g dark chocolate (80% cocoa solids), melted

200g dates, stoned

4 tablespoons hot water

150ml olive or other non-flavoured oil

300g cooked beetroots, drained

2 tablespoons muscovado sugar

3 large free-range eggs

1 tablespoon vanilla paste

2 teaspoons baking powder

4 tablespoons cocoa powder

200g wholemeal self-raising flour

For the topping
300g Greek yoghurt

20g dark chocolate (80% cocoa solids), grated or shaved

1/ Preheat the oven to 200°C/180°C fan/400°F/gas 6 and line 1–2 cupcake trays with 16–18 cupcake cases.

2/ Place a small non-stick saucepan over a medium heat and add the chocolate. Heat for 3–5 minutes, stirring continuously, until melted, then remove from the heat. (If you prefer, you can heat it on medium in a microwave until melted.) Set aside.

3/ Place the dates in a food-processor and add the hot water. Blitz until a paste is formed.

4/ Add the oil, beetroots and sugar and blitz again until combined. Now add the eggs, vanilla and melted dark chocolate and blitz once more. Finally, add the baking powder, cocoa and flour and mix until combined.

5/ Divide the mixture between the cupcake cases, filling them about three-quarters full, and bake in the middle of the oven for 15 minutes or until cooked through.

6/ Leave the cupcakes to cool for 10 minutes before removing from the tray.

7/ Before serving, dollop a tablespoon of yoghurt onto each cupcake, then sprinkle with grated chocolate. The cakes will keep in an airtight container for a couple of days – just wait to top with yoghurt and chocolate until you're ready to serve.

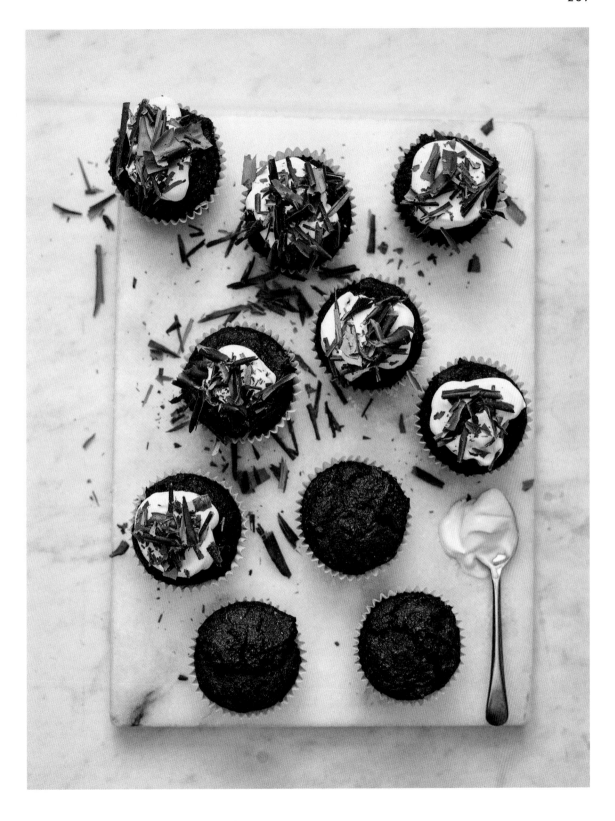

The Ultimate Body Plan for New Mums

quick mixed-berry ripple yoghurt

Prep time:
5 minutes

Calories per serving:
**122 (based on
4 servings)**

A super simple berry yoghurt. You can vary it by changing up the berries you use, but this tried-and-tested combo is a winner in my house.

serves 4–6

140g ripe strawberries, hulled

140g blackberries

500g Greek yoghurt

1 tablespoon runny honey (optional; add if the fruit isn't as ripe as you would like)

1/ Place most of the berries in a bowl (saving a handful for the top), then mash with a fork until they form a paste.

2/ Add half the yoghurt and mix in, then swirl the remaining yoghurt through to create a ripple effect. Serve topped with the remaining berries and a drizzle of honey, if using.

blueberry chia pudding

Not only is this an amazing dessert, but also, weirdly enough, it makes a brilliant breakfast dish! Incredibly easy to make, strangely pretty to look at (so great to serve at a dinner party), and kids love it. Win-win-win.

Prep time:
5 minutes (plus 6 hours chilling)

Calories per serving:
268 (based on 4 servings)

serves 4-6

80g frozen blueberries, plus extra to serve

1 teaspoon vanilla essence

400ml unsweetened fortified almond milk

4 teaspoons Mixed Nut Butter (page 164) or your favourite shop-bought nut butter

½ ripe avocado, peeled and stoned

65g chia seeds

handful of almonds or hazelnuts, roughly chopped

1/ Place the blueberries, vanilla essence, almond milk, nut butter and avocado in a blender and whizz to create a smooth liquid.

2/ Pour the mixture into a large bowl, then stir in the chia seeds.

3/ Cover and leave in the fridge for 5 hours (or overnight) to set. If you choose to leave it overnight, the mixture will be a bit *too* set in the morning, bu you can just stir in a little almond milk to loosen it up.

4/ Divide into serving dishes and top with extra blueberries and a sprinkling of nuts.

fruity crumble

Prep time:
5 minutes

Cooking time:
35 minutes

Calories per serving:
412

This recipe is delicious with any fruit, so clear out your fridge, freezer or fruit bowl and go mad! I recommend you choose at least one stone fruit (like peaches or plums), to stop the dish becoming too liquidy.

serves 6

2 apples, peeled, cored and chopped into 2cm pieces

4 plums, stoned and roughly chopped

150g fresh or frozen raspberries

zest and juice of 1 orange

100g unsalted butter, cold and cubed

100g spelt or wholemeal flour

1 teaspoon ground cinnamon

150g rolled oats

50g dark brown soft sugar

natural yoghurt, to serve

1/ Preheat the oven to 200°C/180°C fan/400°F/gas 6.

2/ Place a saucepan over a medium heat. Add the fruit, along with the orange zest and juice, and cook for a couple of minutes until the fruit is starting to soften.

3/ Meanwhile, place the butter, flour and cinnamon in a large bowl and rub between your thumb and finger to create little crumbs. If you prefer, you can place them in a food-processor and blitz to form a breadcrumb-like texture.

4/ Stir in the oats and sugar. If you were using a food-processor before, transfer the mixture to a bowl now and stir, as you don't want to blitz up the oats.

5/ Pour the fruit into a 20cm round ovenproof dish, then scatter over the crumble topping, making sure all the fruit is covered.

6/ Bake for 30 minutes, or until the top is golden and the fruit is bubbling away and cooked through.

7/ Leave to cool slightly before serving with a spoonful of natural yoghurt or a little custard, because why the hell not, eh?

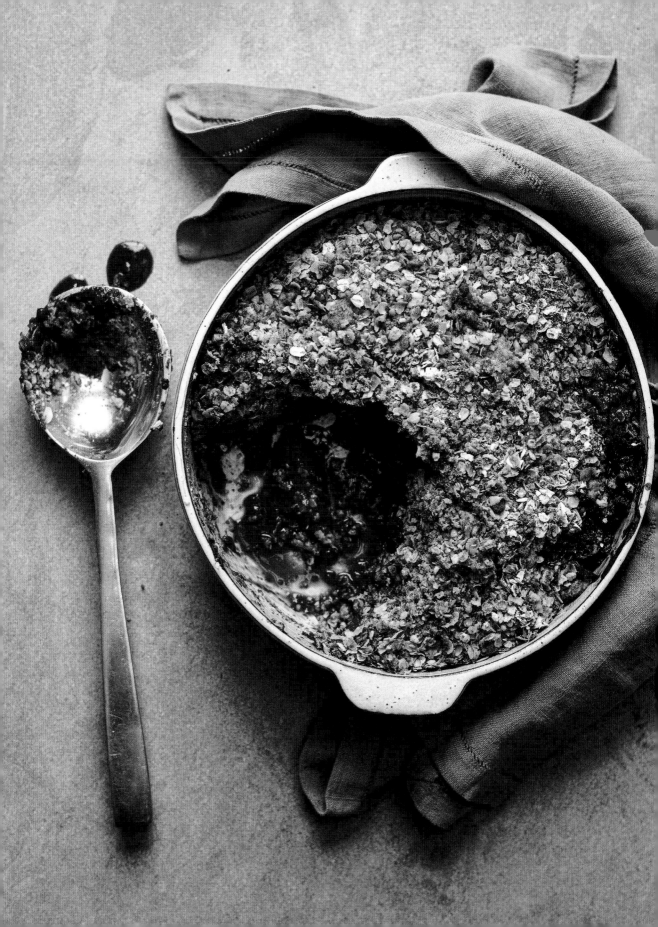

strawberry lollies

Prep time:
5 minutes

Freezing time:
6 hours

Calories per serving:
74

Is there anything better than a lolly when you're hot, bothered and breastfeeding? The answer, friends, is no, there's not. So make your own – it's really easy, and means you'll always have some in the freezer for emergencies.

makes approx. 6 lollies
(depending on mould)

250g fresh strawberries, hulled and halved

200g Greek yoghurt

1 tablespoon runny honey, to sweeten (optional)

1/ Add the strawberries and yoghurt to a blender and blitz until mixed. Taste, adding a little honey if it's not sweet enough, and blitz again.

2/ Pour the mixture into lolly moulds and freeze for at least 6 hours or until totally frozen.

3/ Dish out to your kids, your partner, the neighbours – anyone who either deserves something cool and sweet, or who you'd love to shut up for 5 minutes.

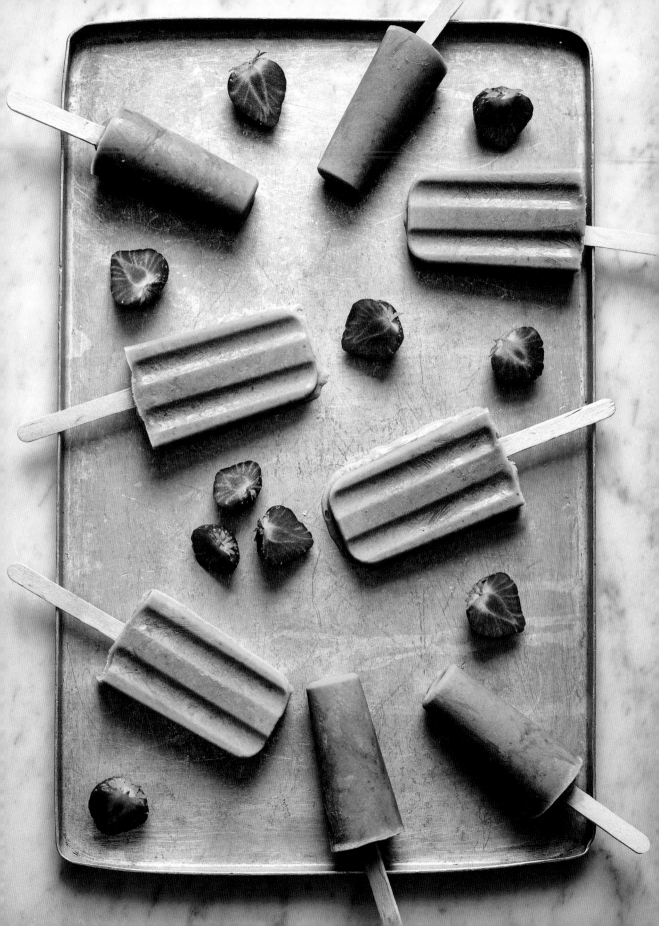

easy raspberry sorbet

Really refreshing and tangy – just like a sorbet should be. Lovely to have after dinner, on a hot day or when you're flat on your back, too tired to move (just ask someone else to get you some).

Prep time:
5 minutes

Freezing time:
4–5 hours

Calories per serving:
37

serves 8

50ml maple syrup or agave syrup

350g frozen raspberries

200ml water

handful of baby mint leaves

1/ Place the maple syrup and raspberries in a food-processor. Add the water and blitz to combine.

2/ Pour the mixture into ice cube trays (you will need a few) or a freezer-proof plastic container and cover.

3/ Freeze for 4–5 hours.

4/ Carefully scoop the frozen mixture out of your chosen container and return it to the food-processor. Pulse to create an icy, slushy texture. Transfer into a freezer-proof plastic container and freeze again, ready to serve whenever you like. Just remove it from the freezer a few minutes before serving to soften a little.

5/ To serve, scoop out into bowls and top with a few mint leaves for added pizazz.

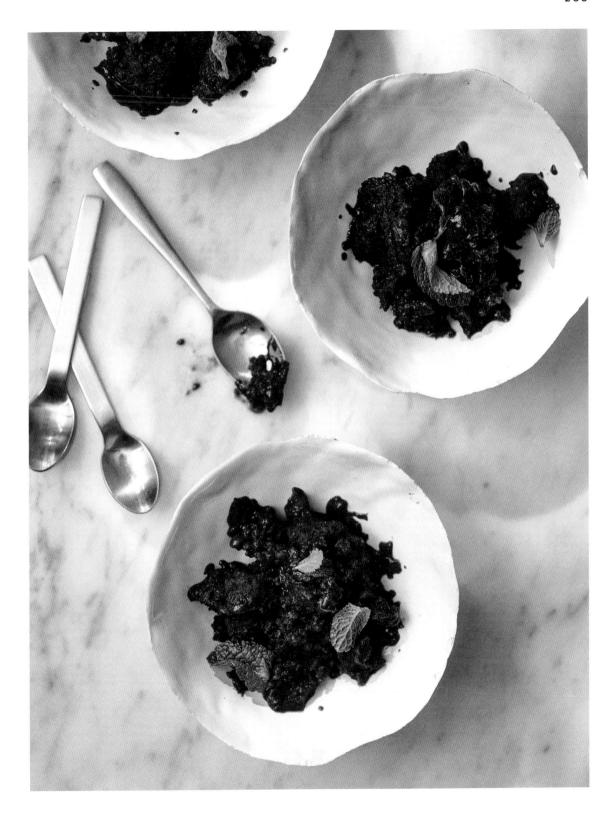

The Ultimate Body Plan for New Mums

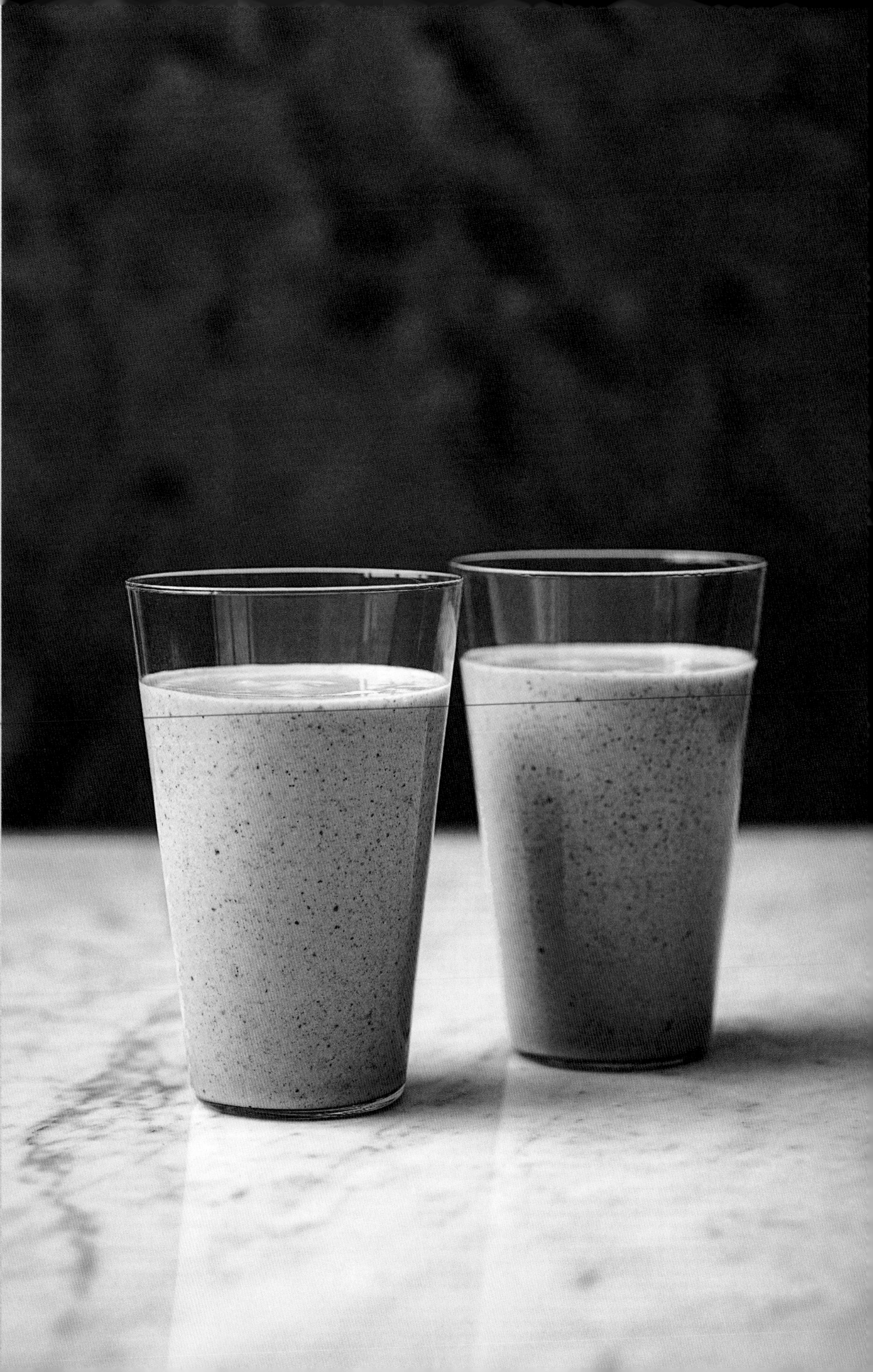

green power smoothie

Prep time:
10 minutes

Calories per serving:
317

This smoothie is great to have post-workout to repair tired muscles. Keeping frozen whole-leaf spinach in the freezer is a game-changer – just add a few balls to smoothies or other dishes for a great source of iron (it doesn't need to be defrosted first for this recipe). You can also add a scoop of protein powder or ground nuts for an added protein boost if needed. Note: the calorie information given here is based on the version with nuts and honey, not protein powder.

serves 2

50g frozen spinach

80g (about 3 florets) frozen cauliflower

½ avocado, peeled and stoned

1 ripe banana, halved

a handful of nuts (or, if you need an extra boost, 1 scoop of protein powder)

1 tablespoon runny honey (if not using protein powder)

400ml coconut water or unsweetened fortified almond milk

1/ Simply throw the spinach, cauliflower, avocado and banana into a large blender.

2/ Add the nuts and honey (or protein powder, if using), along with the coconut water or almond milk. Blend it all together until combined.

3/ Serve and chug it down. If you're not sharing with someone else, you can save the second portion for another day. It will keep for 1–2 days in the fridge – just blitz it up again before drinking.

watermelon refresher

Prep time:
5 minutes

Calories per serving:
77

Fresh watermelon blitzed with coconut water is the most refreshing drink of all time (I'll fight you on this). Neck a glass in the morning for a really positive, go-getting start to the day. It also makes great lollies.

serves 2

250g ice cubes

250g watermelon chunks

250ml coconut water

4 sprigs of mint, plus extra to serve

1/ Place all the ingredients in a blender and blitz to combine.

2/ Divide between 2 glasses and serve with a few extra sprigs of mint and a (non-plastic) straw!

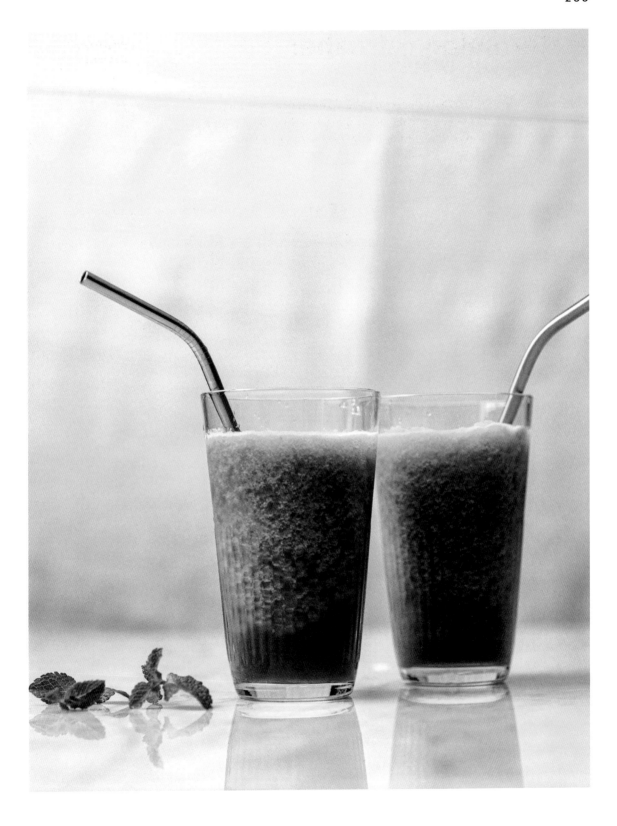

citrus cooler

Prep time:
5 minutes

Calories per serving:
**47 (based on
4 servings)**

This is perfect for when you're craving a fizzy drink after a bad night. Not only does it hydrate, the sour tang also properly wakes you up. Freestyling with ingredients is encouraged: pomegranate works nicely (and gives it an amazing vivid colour) while grapefruit is ideal for lip-smacking eyes-wide-open zing.

serves 4–6

a good few handfuls of ice

1 lemon, zest peeled into strips and juiced

2 limes, zest peeled into strips and juiced

2 oranges, zest peeled into strips and juiced

250ml coconut water

1 tablespoon maple syrup

1¾ pints sparkling water

1/ Place the ice in a large jug. Add the lemon, lime and orange juice and strips of zest, along with the coconut water and maple syrup.

2/ Top up with the sparkling water and serve: perfect for a hot summer's day.

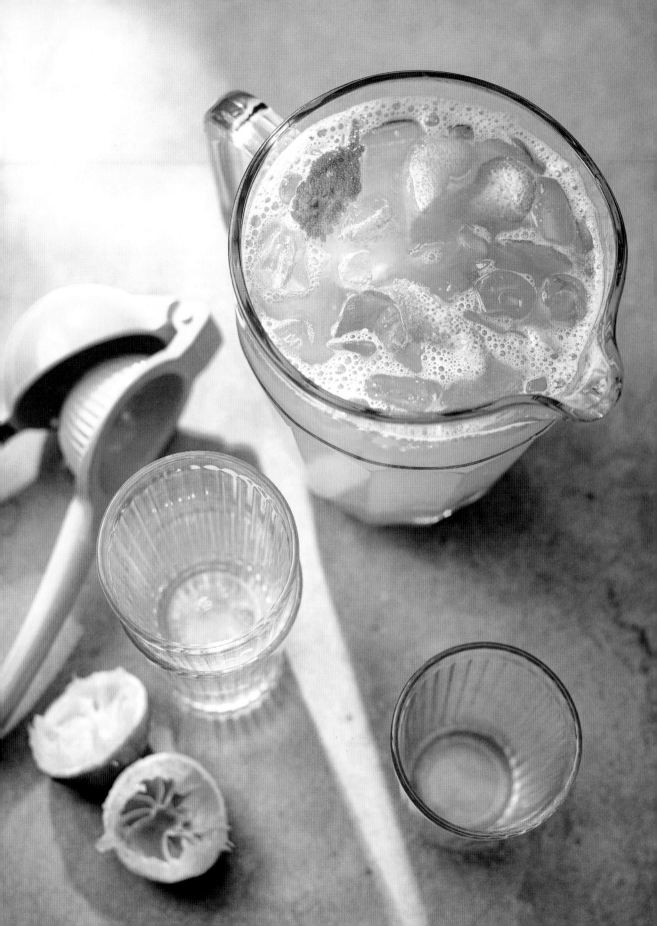

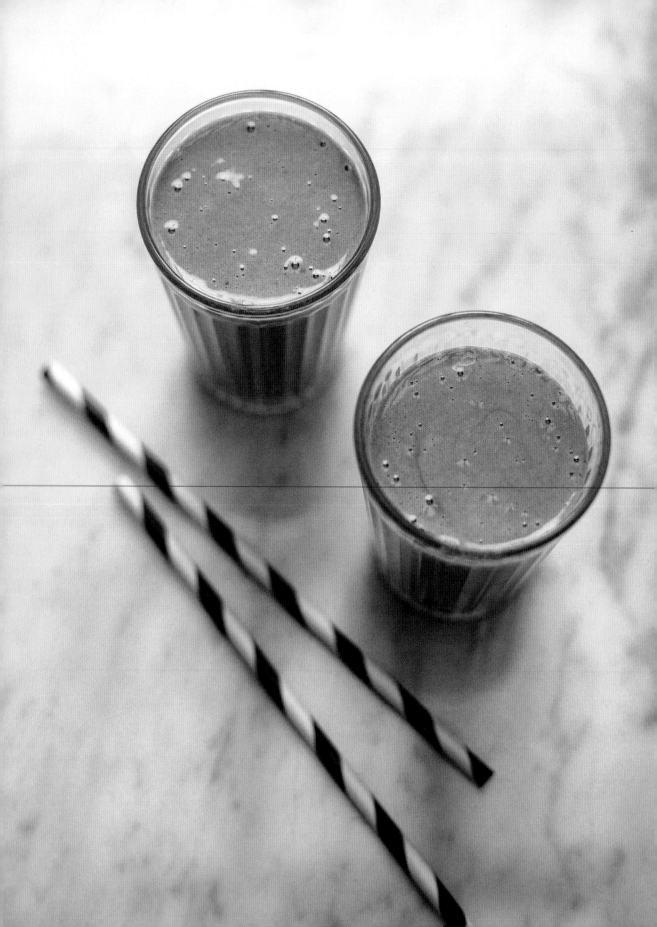

banana & chocolate milkshake

Prep time:
5 minutes

Calories per serving:
213

This is a perfect alternative to grabbing a chocolatey snack mid-afternoon. If you drink normal milk, go for that, but if you use dairy alternatives, stick to unsweetened or fortified oat, almond or soy milk.

serves 2

200ml unsweetened fortified oat milk

200g frozen banana

1 tablespoon cocoa powder

30g rolled oats

1/ Add everything to a blender and blitz until combined.

2/ Serve immediately. (If you have any left over, pour it into ice lolly moulds and save for a hot day or for the kids as a 'treat' for pudding.)

beetroot & berry booster

Prep time:
2 minutes

Calories per serving:
152

You'll need a good blender to really break the beetroot down (no one wants a drink with beetroot chunks in it). If you prefer a creamier texture, you can add some milk.

serves 2

a few ice cubes

250ml coconut water

100g cooked beetroot

100g frozen blueberries

½ avocado, peeled, stoned and sliced

juice of ½ lemon

1 teaspoon milled flaxseed

1/ Place all the ingredients in a high-speed blender and blitz until combined and smooth.

2/ Drink immediately, or, if you want to make it in advance, keep in the fridge for up to 1 day, and then blitz again or stir well before serving.

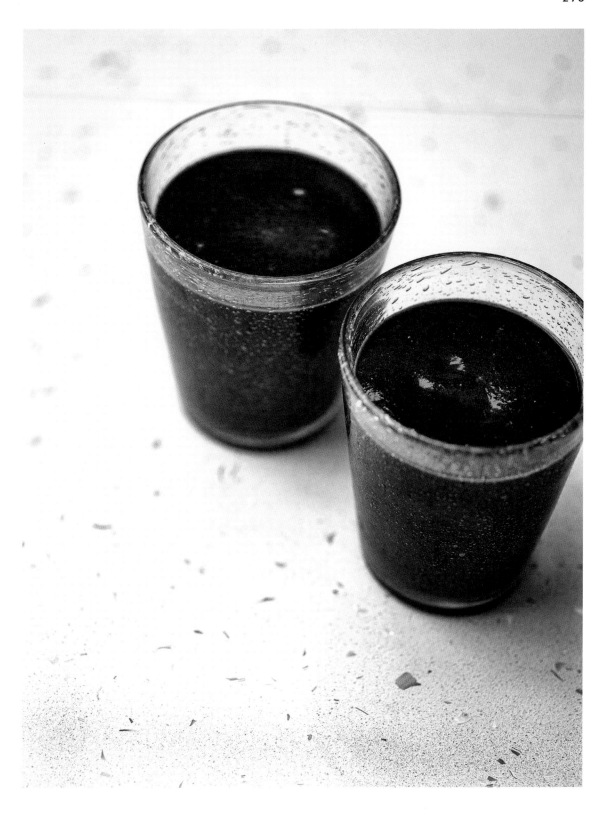

The Ultimate Body Plan for New Mums

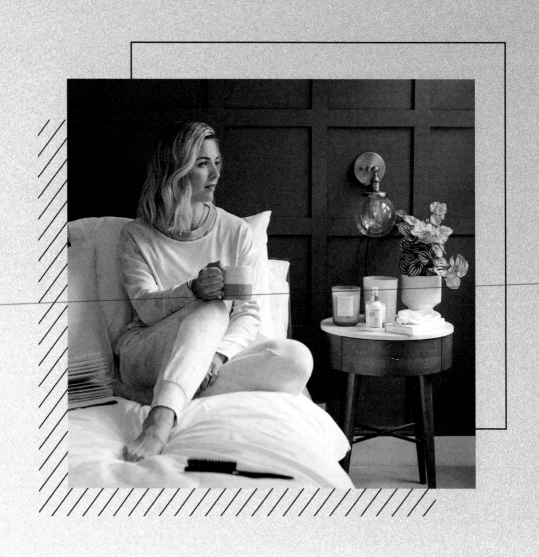

WELLBEING

IT'S ALL WELL & GOOD

I really wanted to include a wellbeing section in this book because having a baby knocks you on your arse – both physically and mentally – and so I think it's essential to address all aspects of self-care. If your mental health is all over the shop, you're not going to feel like eating well or working out. In just the same way, if you're not eating well or working out, it can make you feel like crap mentally. It's all connected.

I know that wellbeing and self-care can seem like buzzwords, or trendy topics to sound knowledgeable about at parties ('Oh, yes, I've practised chanting for years. I can't believe you've never tried it,' etc.). But the fact that everyone's talking about how to look after yourself is a great thing! It means there's a shift in public acceptance about the importance of prioritising our mental health – that it's not something to be embarrassed about or to hide away from. I get why you might be tempted to roll your eyes though – particularly when every Tom, Dick and Harry seems to know a new trick or shortcut to feeling better. It's hard to know who or what to trust. That's why all of the tips you'll find in this section are my own personal recommendations – things that have worked for me. No hocus-pocus or 'my mate Dave's aunt once did this and it changed her life'.

It's not 'woo-woo' or tree-huggy to want to make sure you're in the right headspace to look after your family. It's essential! These tips will help you to relax, recharge and

These strategies are intended to help you with the day-to-day challenges of motherhood and self-care. If you feel like you're really struggling and/or may be suffering from depression or generalised anxiety disorder, please speak to your GP about getting further help.

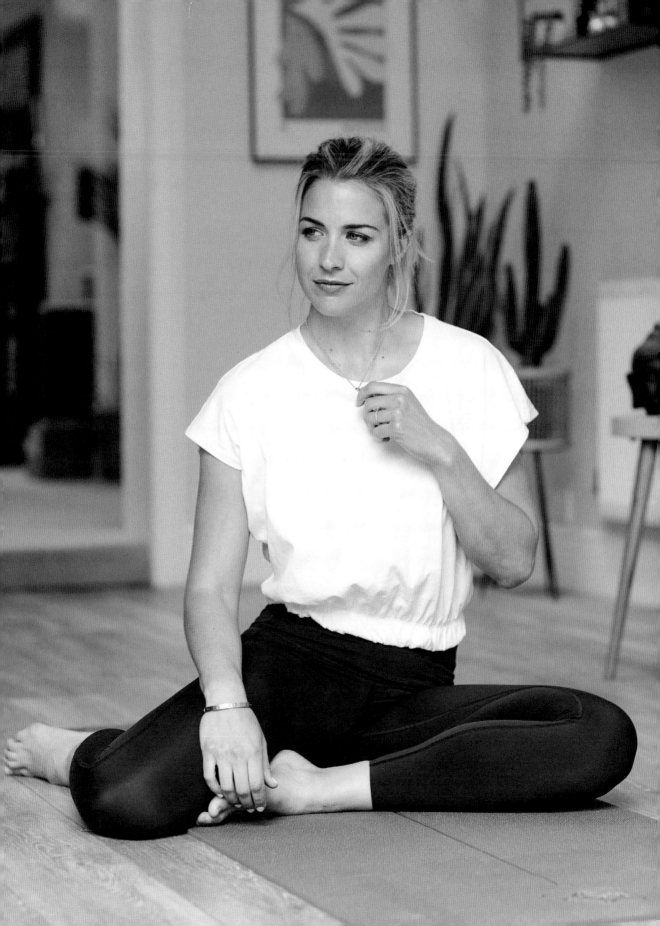

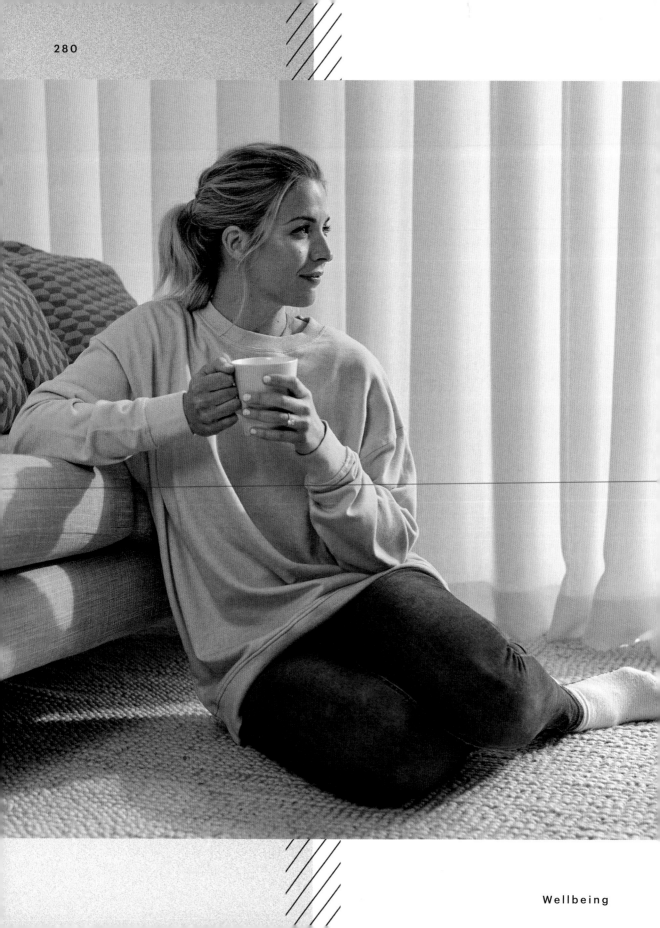

reset, boosting self-esteem with the goal of feeling energised and confident. We all experience down days and we all have particular patterns of behaviour that we find ourselves defaulting to. Paying attention to your thoughts and behaviour – and giving yourself the space and time to do so – will enable you to recognise when you're storming off down well-worn negative paths. Our thoughts affect our behaviour, and vice versa. Tuning into that is so important when your life's been turned upside down.

In this book, I have avoided mentioning the pandemic and lockdown for various reasons, but it's the MASSIVE tap-dancing elephant in the room. We've all just been through something unprecedented and will continue to deal with the fallout for decades. And, to have also become a new parent during this time? How completely bizarre! Talk about dealing with change! Everyone's usual support system was essentially outlawed. Dealing with a new baby during this time was a mammoth task – and you did it! You freaking did it! That's not something to be taken lightly. So please make time for yourself in your calendar. You deserve it. Make it official, prioritising it like you would a business meeting. And, once you get into a wellbeing routine, you'll gradually notice you feel better, stronger and more able to deal with stuff. So do some chanting (page 288), put on that Superwoman tee (page 282), scream 'OMG, WHAT THE HELL IS HAPPENING?!', into the abyss, and I'll see you at the gym (pages 54–131).

Make time for yourself in your calendar. You deserve it. Make it official, prioritising it like you would a business meeting.

EVERYDAY SELF-CARE

These simple practices always make me feel more with-it and like I have a better handle on the day. It's about acknowledging that I need a moment, that I deserve some love and that looking after myself matters.

1/ DRINK A GLASS OF WATER IMMEDIATELY UPON WAKING UP

This is almost laughably simple and yet makes such a difference! Drinking a glass of water kicks your digestive system into gear, automatically making you feel more alert physically – and therefore mentally. Such an easy win.

2/ PULL ON SOME CLEAN CLOTHES (OR, BETTER YET, SOME 'POWER GEAR')

It may feel like a waste to put on clean clothes when they're only going to get puked on, but a fresh outfit can feel like a fresh start. Also, what we wear has been proven to change how we view ourselves. In a study, people who were asked to wear a Superman T-shirt rated themselves as more likeable – and even physically stronger – as a result! So pull on that damn Superwoman (ahem) tee, because that's what you are. Yes, even with puke down your back.

3/ BRUSH YOUR HAIR AND PUT ON SOME MOISTURISER

Funny how we can spend fifteen minutes arranging our kid's hair into adorable pigtails but won't brush our own mops for weeks. Just spritzing some dry shampoo on your barnet and slathering on some moisturiser or eye cream can act as a mental signal to yourself that you're 'getting ready' (plus your tired skin has probably been crying out for moisturiser). Who cares if no one will see you but the postman? You're doing it for you.

4/ SET A POSITIVE AFFIRMATION TO PING UP ONCE A DAY ON YOUR PHONE

Either choose an affirmation from the list opposite, invent your own or add an old fave. Whatever you choose, though, make sure it pops up during a typically stressful moment of the day. Nothing gives me a lift like having a message appear saying, 'You're doing better than you think you are,' when I'm trying to navigate complete chaos.

5/ MAKE YOURSELF A LITTLE SANCTUARY

In the madness of new parenthood, your baby and all their stuff can take over your home. We're so eager to carve out some space for them, we forget about our own needs. Creating a 'nook' for yourself can be a real mental boost. This might be a special chair with an uninterrupted view of the outside world, or a quiet spot where beautiful morning light hits – anywhere will do! (I've kept the chair I used to go and escape on after I had Mia. I'm so attached to it that I had it reupholstered when we moved to a new house so it would match the new stuff.) Your sanctuary is 'your' place, and so it should be baby-free. Make a rule that you only go there when you're having time to yourself, and aim for at least five quiet minutes there once a day.

6/ DO THE THINGS YOU ENJOYED BEFORE HAVING A BABY

Just because you've had a baby doesn't mean you suddenly don't like going to the cinema, seeing your friends, going on city breaks or dancing like a loon to nineties garage tunes. Scheduling these things – with or without your baby – will remind you that you are still you. My mates and I try to get together for a baby-free lunch or night out at least once every six weeks. Not a lot, I know, but that makes me look forward to them even more.

7/ DROP YOUR SHOULDERS, LIFT YOUR CHIN AND STRAIGHTEN YOUR BACK

Do it right now. Studies have shown that simply amending our posture can make us feel more confident. Sitting or standing up straight makes us feel more go-getting. We often hunch over and curl in on ourselves when we're stressed without even realising it, so adjusting your posture in this way can help you tune in to your body and therefore your mind. It's a way of taking back control.

10 positive affirmations for whenever you need a lift

1/ Taking care of myself makes me a better mum.

2/ They're not stretch marks, they're tiger stripes – and I'm the Queen of the Jungle!

3/ I don't need to 'get my body back'. It didn't go anywhere – it just changed and adapted to do something incredible.

4/ My body had a baby; it can manage a sodding workout.

5/ Even on my down days, my baby thinks I'm the best person in the whole world.

6/ Everyone feels like a total fraud sometimes.

7/ *'Being a mother is learning about strengths you didn't know you had, and dealing with fears you didn't know existed.'* – Linda Wooten, *A Mother's Thoughts*

8/ I've got through all of my worst days before and I'm still here.

9/ *'Worrying is like riding a rocking horse – it's something to do, but it gets you nowhere.'* – My dad.

10/ It's no one's job to be perfect: it's about being persistent. Small steps will still get you there.

TALK
IT OUT

One of the biggest surprises for me after having Mia was how jealous I felt about Gorka's freedom. It can seem massively unfair that, purely because of biology, the woman takes the brunt of, well, everything to do with the early days of parenting.

It's our body, our hormones and our boobs (if you're breastfeeding) that do all of the work. Meanwhile, our partners can eat what they want, drink what they want and pick up exactly where they left off. They don't have farty-smelling cabbage leaves stuck down their bras, nor do they have to slide down the stairs on their arses so as not to tear their scars.

As I've already mentioned, Gorka had to go on tour soon after I'd given birth. It wasn't ideal, but it was a contractual commitment and we'd both known it would happen. What I hadn't bargained for, though, was my bubbling resentment. I think it was probably exacerbated by the fact that Gorka's job is so physical and represented everything I couldn't do. He wasn't only out there working – he was bloody dancing! It's almost funny. Like someone can-canning past you when you can't get off the sofa. (Obvs he never did that, but imagining him doing so now is making me chuckle.)

As I explained earlier, it was only after I told him how I was feeling that I realised he also felt out of whack. Not only was he missing us both hugely, but also he was struggling to find his feet in his role as a new dad. Other halves can feel like a spare prick at a wedding when a baby's first born. The mother-and-baby bond is already forged before birth, as we've felt the kicks, hiccups and rib punches during the last few months of carrying them. Partners have to work at building their connection with the baby, while also finding themselves on the sharp end of our mood swings, exhaustion, frustration and fear.

My advice is to simply talk to each other. Effective communication can be the first thing to go when you're knackered and emotional, which is why it's so important to chat about things before they boil over. Book in some time alone just to be with each other. Cook a meal together, grab a takeaway, watch a serial-killer documentary – anything to re-establish a bond, have a laugh (or scream if you choose the serial-killer doc option) and get some time and space to just be. If you're a single parent, talk about how you're feeling with a family member, friend, colleague or expert. Don't suffer in silence: it won't do you any good, and this has the knock-on effect of not doing your baby any good, either.

HERE ARE SOME GOOD CONVERSATIONAL TRICKS I USE TO TALK ABOUT MY FEELINGS WITHOUT CAUSING UNNECESSARY FRICTION:

- **DON'T GO IN WITH AN ACCUSATORY 'YOU'.** By this, I mean phrases like 'you do this' or 'you don't do that'. Instead, try to work around it, making it a 'we' conversation: 'It feels as if there's a bit of a bad vibe in the house at the moment. What can we do to sort it? Can we talk about it?' or even, 'Can I hand over control of bath time tonight? Two nights on the trot and I'm shattered.' That automatically feels less angry than, 'YOU HAVEN'T DONE ANY BATH TIMES, YOU LAZY GIT.'

- **AVOID THE WORDS 'NEVER' AND 'ALWAYS'.** For example, try not to say things like 'you *never* do this' or 'you *always* do that'. It's rarely true that someone 'always' or 'never' does anything, and so they'll be able to come up with instances of when they did do it – which isn't the point! You'll end up arguing over minutiae and not getting to the actual problem. Instead, stick only to the facts.

- **REMEMBER: OPINIONS AREN'T FACTS.** If you're feeling particularly livid, have a word with yourself before letting rip and work out whether you're angry at something factual or something you've just made up in your head. For example, imagine you want to say: 'You don't fancy me anymore.' That's not a fact – it's very definitely an opinion. You can't read your partner's mind, yet you're telling them how they feel as if it's a cast-iron truth. They'd be well within their rights to call that out as 'FAKE NEWS!'. However, if you simply stick 'I feel like' in front of it, it's factual (you do feel that way) and you're getting to the heart of the matter: 'I feel like you don't fancy me anymore.' They can't argue with how you feel, or be annoyed that you're trying to address it, and you're being honest – with them and yourself – when you tell them you feel a bit insecure and in need of some reassurance and affection.

GETTING SOME SLEEEEEEP

Sleep? 'What's that?' I hear you cry. Fair question. Don't worry, I'm not going to try to tell you how to get your baby to sleep (ha! Even writing that made me laugh), but I am going to recommend a few tricks that can help *you* to drop off, if and when you're ever allowed to.

Sleep is when your body not only recovers from the day just gone, but also sets itself up for the day ahead. Lack of sleep (as you'll be well aware by now) can affect everything: your mood, energy levels, motivation and appetite. Not getting enough kip affects the hormones leptin and ghrelin, which monitor appetite. This is why you'll feel hungrier and eat more when you're tired (because you're unable to recognise when you're full). You'll also make worse food choices, as you're knackered, can't be bothered to cook and crave a quick sugar hit. Additionally, you'll feel far less inclined to train and, when you do, your recovery times will suffer, as your muscles recuperate during sleep. So, both more sleep and better-quality sleep are the goal. Here are some things that can help:

01/ MAKE SURE YOU HAVE A GOOD MATTRESS

If sleep is a problem for you anyway, having an uncomfortable, flea-laden, dust-ridden mattress is not going to help matters. Mattresses tend to pass their sell-by-date every ten years, but if you're waking up aching and sore, if it's visibly damaged, if you think it may be contributing to allergies, or if it's still uncomfortable after you've flipped it over, it's time for a new one.

02/ KEEP IT COOL

Sleep prefers cold temperatures to hot ones. When the body reaches a deeper level of sleep, your core body temperature drops. A hot room can hike it up again, disrupting the quality of rest you get. So, instead of keeping your whole bedroom hot, keep it cool, and invest in a bigger duvet, wear bed socks (your feet get colder than the rest of your body) or have a hot-water bottle to keep things cosy.

03/ DON'T LOOK AT YOUR PHONE OR COMPUTER IN THE HOUR BEFORE BEDTIME

The blue light emitted from the screens decreases melatonin, the 'sleepy hormone'. Read a book, listen to music, watch the TV or do a puzzle instead.

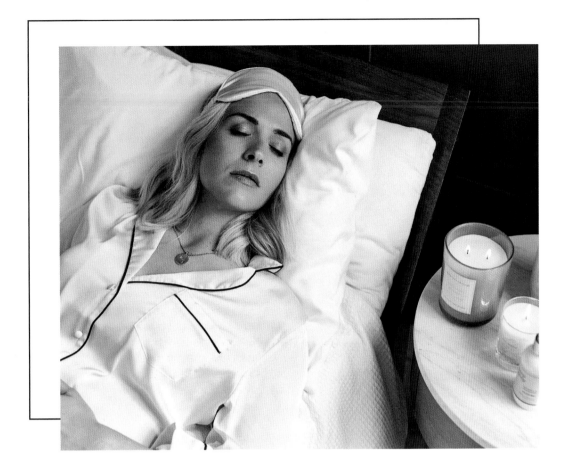

04/ DON'T DRINK CAFFEINE IN THE FOUR TO SIX HOURS BEFORE YOU WANT TO TRY TO SLEEP

Alcohol, too, will lead to disrupted and fragmented sleep (hello, 3 a.m. beer fear!), as will, perhaps strangely, smoking. Nicotine arouses your nervous system, and increases your respiratory rate and blood pressure – none of which is conducive to snoozing. So, have a deadline for caffeine per day (see page 141), lay off the booze while trying to get into a sleep routine (you shouldn't be drinking while on the plan anyway) and quit those cigs.

05/ USE AN APP TO MONITOR YOUR SLEEP

When tired, we have a tendency to exaggerate how bad it is, saying, 'I haven't had a wink's sleep in months.' Being able to see that we actually got four or five hours, while not ideal, can be quite reassuring.

06/ POUR A FEW DROPS OF LAVENDER OIL ON YOUR PILLOW OR INVEST IN A LAVENDER DIFFUSER

Lavender has been relied upon for centuries by people looking to reduce stress and relax.

SELF-CARE TECHNIQUES TO TRY

Chant with me

OK, bear with me here. On YouTube you can find videos of Tina Turner performing several 'Nam-Myōhō-Renge-Kyō' chants. Nam-Myōhō-Renge-Kyō is an essential part of Nichiren Buddhism. The phrase sums up the principal underlying Buddhist beliefs (that's the most simplistic description ever so I highly recommend giving it a google if you'd like more information) and chanting it is a way for believers to channel positivity and inner power from within. It's a way of finding peace in a meditative state.

How did I come across it? From *Soapstar Superstar*, as mad as that sounds! I appeared on the ITV show in 2007, and my vocal coach recommended chanting to soothe my nerves. I would get so nervous before I went on stage that my hands would shake and I'd feel sweat pooling in the small of my back. 'I can't do this,' I'd whisper, genuinely considering whether I could leg it out of the nearest exit without anyone noticing. During a vocal session at her house, my coach asked if I'd ever done any chanting. 'No, I'm not a hippy,' I laughed. But she was dead serious. She introduced me to the Nam-Myōhō-Renge-Kyō chant, and I can't tell you how much it relaxed me. It didn't only calm me down, it unblocked my nose, cleared my airways and made me feel stronger. We only did it for three minutes each time, and I remember thinking, 'What is this – magic?!' You may be familiar with chanting if you practised hypnobirthing, as it's a common strategy used to keep mums-to-be calm during contractions.

I found a couple of chanting videos online featuring monks, but they were a bit too intense for me. And then I discovered Tina Turner's videos. Total game-changer! I love Tina! Now I practise with her for a couple of minutes in the morning, before bed or whenever I'm very nervous. It's all about your breath – taking deep anchoring breaths. You have to really focus on your breathing in order to be able to get the words out, which is very meditative and mindful. The repetitions, the chimes and the deep tonality mean you completely lose yourself and zone out. It's actually incredibly beautiful. You go into yourself and create your own little world – it always makes me feel quite emotional. I highly recommend suspending your cynicism like I did and giving it a go.

Throw the baby out with the bathwater...

...and get in the tub yourself. Oh, I do like a bath. Showers are for getting clean and starting your day, but baths are pure luxury. The first time my mum and stepdad had Mia overnight, Gorka and I were like, 'Right! What shall we do?! Go to the pub or a restaurant?' In the end, we ordered a takeaway, then I put on a face mask and had a bath while Gorka watched the football: absolute bliss! Having a bath feels so decadent – bubbles in, music on, conking out. Speak to your health visitor about when it's safe for you to be in the tub (and investigate 'sitz baths', which are specially designed to help heal the perineal area postpartum). As soon as you're given the green light, slide in and imbibe some of these well-documented health benefits:

- Getting into hot water can improve blood circulation (and oxygenate the blood) as your heart beats faster.

- The steam can clear sinuses.

- Taking the time to soak in the bath can calm you, helping you feel 'quieter' and more relaxed.

- The warmth and relaxation encourage you to breathe more deeply and slowly, making you feel more meditative, and easing tension and fatigue.

- A bath can help with muscle soreness and tension, especially if you add Epsom salts, a naturally occurring salt product. Put 300g in your bathwater and bathe for at least fifteen minutes to feel the benefit.

- The warm water can soothe the episiotomy repair and ease swollen haemorrhoids after birth.

Jump on the yoga bandwagon

There's nothing negative or stressful about yoga. Every pose, every breath, every movement is beneficial for body and mind. It's a great feeling. Even if you only get in a ten-minute session, you know that that was a good ten minutes. I think practising yoga is one of the kindest things you can do for your body: you're allowing it to stretch, move, breathe and relax. You're giving it – every bit of it! – the attention it deserves. Yoga makes you concentrate on parts of your body that usually go completely ignored, like your feet and wrists. You tune in to your muscles and breathe into them. It's a fantastic way of getting out of your head, because you really have to focus on completing the movements properly. I highly recommend finding a local class – it's a great way to meet people and get some personal advice. However, there are brill online tutorials, too. I started by simply googling 'beginner's yoga' and quickly found a load of options with sessions ranging from ten to fifty minutes.

Lose yourself in a good book

I'm a massive reader. I always have been, ever since I was a little girl. (*The Tiger Who Came to Tea* and *The Worst Witch* series were my favourite books growing up. On Thursday nights, my grandma would come for tea, and she'd always read them to me before bed). Nowadays, I try to read for at least fifteen minutes each night (usually while Gorka watches his Spanish TV shows), and my go-to books are biographies of people I admire, or non-fiction books about topics I find interesting. I want to learn! I love feeling inspired by other people's achievements and learning more about their philosophies on life. Reading is also soothing, and a great thing to do to force us off our phones (especially before bed!).

Below are some books I've read recently that I highly recommend:

- *Peak 40* by Dr Marc Bubbs. This is so good! It's about how best to prepare the body, both mentally and physically, for the changes you'll experience when you hit forty.

- *Greenlights* by Matthew McConaughey. You can't help but read this in his voice! It's full of great life affirmations and positivity, plus funny insider stories about Hollywood.

- *The Body Book* by Cameron Diaz. This was released in 2013, but I still dig it out sometimes for a bit of inspo. It's all about the ageing process, about going through it naturally and learning to appreciate our bodies at different stages of life. It's essentially about working with ageing instead of fighting against it — which I'm all for.

- *My Fight/Your Fight* by Ronda Rousey. I'm a huge Ronda fan — it's down to her that we have a female division in UFC (Ultimate Fighting Championship) today. She had a tough start in life (from dealing with academic problems to having to cope with her father's suicide when she was just eight years old), yet she continuously worked to better herself, always making changes and striving for more — breaking some world records along the way. Anyone will feel motivated by her success story.

Set achievable goals

Having goals is admirable. They give us purpose and hope, and shove us out of our comfort zones. Being specific about what you want to achieve will make you far more likely to get out there and do it than if you just have some vague idea that you might, possibly, maybe, one day want to give that thing a go. You just have to make sure you don't fall into that far-too-common trap of setting yourself up for a fall. That happens when you try to do too much, too soon, and set yourself unrealistic targets.

I did an interview for a magazine recently, during which the journalist told me, 'I have three sugars in my tea – and I drink a lot of tea every day. I know it's unhealthy, but I can't stop.'

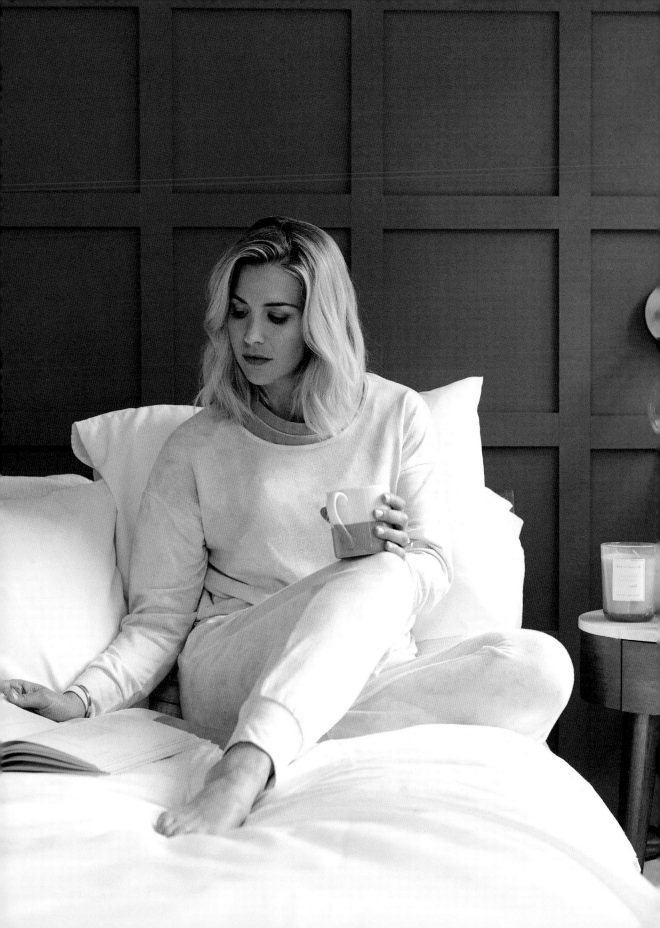

I told her, 'Rather than cut it out, make it an elimination process. So this week, tell yourself, "I'm going to have two sugars rather than three."'

'Yeah,' she said, 'but two's still bad!'

I said, 'Yes – but it's not as bad as three, is it?!'

If she manages to go down to two sugars that week, she can try one the next week – and so on.

We often try to ban ourselves from doing stuff completely – going cold turkey. Or we might introduce something all-consuming into our lives immediately, with no easing in. The all-or-nothing route rarely (if ever) works. It's like setting yourself the goal of running a marathon in three months' time when you've never finished a 5km run, or aiming to become a top-class chef in just six months when you currently can't nail beans on toast. Running a marathon and becoming a chef are really worthy goals, but why put yourself under such huge amounts of pressure? The training and learning are part of the journey. It's why the training part of this plan is designed to be completed in phases that gradually increase in difficulty. Taking things step-by-step is the only way of reaching your goal properly, safely and enjoyably. If you were planning on climbing Mount Everest, you'd strategise for months (if not years). You'd have to do all the training, get all the gear, plan everything down to the last detail – and then spend three weeks actually climbing the damn mountain! It's not like someone says, 'Hey, fancy giving Everest a bash tomorrow?' and everyone's like, 'Sure – done.'

You can still plan to climb Everest; you just have to be realistic and smart about it. Which leads me neatly to this SMART acronym – an easy way to structure goal-making. Simply ask yourself: 'Is my goal...'

... **specific?** My goal needs to be well-defined and clear. What exactly do I want to achieve?

... **measurable?** How will I know when I've completed it?

... **achievable?** Do I have the resources I need to complete it?

... **realistic?** Is my goal within reach and relevant?

... **timely?** Have I put in a (realistic) timeline for achieving my goal?

Here are some examples so you can see how this kind of goal-setting works.

GOAL	SPECIFIC	MEASUREABLE	ACHIEVABLE	REALISTIC	TIMELY
I want to meet more new mums.	I will join a local mum and baby group.	I have to sign up and attend at least one session.	Yes. I can look up groups online and am available two days a week.	Yes.	I will aim to sign up within one week, and go to a session within a fortnight.
I want to feel fitter and stronger.	I want to complete this training programme.	When I finish Phase 3 of the plan.	Yes. I have the book and the kit, and am determined to see it through.	Yes. I'm nervous, but there's no reason I can't do this.	I'm aiming for twelve weeks, but it may take longer and I'm OK with that. I'd like to be on Phase 3 within twenty weeks, though.

It can be useful to break your bigger-picture goals down into smaller steps and use the SMART technique on them. For instance, in the example above, you could treat 'look up mother and baby groups online' as a smaller goal in its own right, and give it its own individual deadline, etc. This approach can help make bigger, long-term goals feel more achievable, and means you can tick each step off your to-do list as you go along (always satisfying).

The point is to enjoy the journey. Pat yourself on the back every step of the way rather than focusing solely on the end result and then kicking yourself if you don't make it. By enjoying the process, you're already succeeding.

CONGRATULATIONS!

Phew! Congratulations on completing *The Ultimate Body Plan for New Mums*! Do your giddy little awkward mum dance right now! This is a massive achievement. I hope you've come out the other side feeling stronger, fitter, healthier and happier.

As I've mentioned throughout the book, how you feel physically is intrinsically linked to how you feel mentally, and vice versa, so looking after your body should have a big impact on your feelings of self-worth and self-belief.

This plan was never about reaching a goal weight. It was about learning how to look after yourself and feel like you again. There will have been points where you gave up, sacrificed training for sleeping (I don't blame you) and dismissed it all as a load of crap meant for 'other people' (perhaps the kind of people who live in a parallel universe with more hours in the day and more motivation). I am so proud that you pushed through the doubts and carried on – and you should be incredibly proud of yourself, too.

At the start of the plan, I asked you to fill out the Motivation Table (page 49), being honest about your goals, motivations and worries. I'd like you to complete another table now, at the end of the journey, as a means to reflect on how far you've come.

Your answers should stand as a testament to what you've had to do to get here: you've overcome self-doubt, made sacrifices, navigated obstacles – and sweated for England! Well done! However, if the table doesn't reflect the kind of change you were hoping for, don't worry – there's no time restriction to this plan. Twelve weeks is just a guideline, giving you the starting blocks for a lifestyle overhaul. Stick with it! Make a conscious decision to persevere, stay motivated and work hard. If you've struggled, that's not a failure. It's a jumping-off point to start recalculating how to make fitness, nutrition and self-care work for you. Don't get despondent – get creative. Remember, everything you've done and are doing sets an example for your little one to follow suit. The same goes for those who have finished and enjoyed the process: keep going! My first twelve-week transformation was five years ago, and I've never looked back. There's no reason to stop now. This is the start of a journey that can last a lifetime.

Thank you for your faith in me, the process and, most of all, yourself. You are one badass parent!

This is only the beginning!

Gemma
xxx

Reflection Table

Date you finished the plan	
How do you feel about having completed the plan?	
Did you reach the goals you listed in your Motivation Table? Did these objectives change during the journey?	
Do you feel stronger and healthier physically?	
Do you feel stronger and healthier mentally?	
What did you most enjoy experiencing during the process? (And did that surprise you?)	
What did you least enjoy? (And did that surprise you?)	
What were the biggest stumbling blocks or obstacles you faced?	
Were you proud of how you navigated those obstacles? Do you think it has made you feel more confident about dealing with issues in other aspects of your life?	
Do you still want the same reward you promised yourself at the start? When are you going to gift it to yourself?	
Rate how you feel about yourself now, on a scale of 1–10 (with 1 being 'I don't like myself' and 10 being 'I'm basically Xena Warrior Princess').	

INDEX

RECIPE INDEX

CONVERSION CHART

Weight conversions

5g	⅛ oz
10g	¼oz
15g	½oz
25/30g	1oz
40g	1½oz
50g	1¾oz
55g	2oz
70g	2½oz
85g	3oz
100g	3½oz
115g	4oz
150g	5½oz
200g	7oz
225g	8oz
250g	9oz
300g	10½oz
350g	12oz
375g	13oz
400g	14oz
450g	1lb
500g	1lb 2oz
600g	1lb 5oz
750g	1lb 10oz
900g	2lb
1kg	2lb 4oz

Volume conversions (liquids)

5ml	–	1 teaspoon
15ml	½fl oz	1 tablespoon
30ml	1fl oz	2 tablespoon
60ml	2fl oz	¼ cup
75ml	2½fl oz	⅓ cup
120ml	4fl oz	½ cup
150ml	5fl oz	⅔ cup
175ml	6fl oz	¾ cup
250ml	8fl oz	1 cup
350ml	12fl oz	1½ cups
500ml	18fl oz	2 cups
1 litre	1¾ pints	4 cups

Volume conversions
(dry ingredients – an approximate guide)

Flour	125g	1 cup
Butter	225g	1 cup (*2 sticks*)
Breadcrumbs (*dried*)	125g	1 cup
Nuts	125g	1 cup
Seeds	160g	1 cup
Dried fruit	150g	1 cup
Dried pulses (*large*)	175g	1 cup
Grains and small dried pulses	200g	1 cup

Length

1cm	½ inch
2.5cm	1 inch
3cm	1¼ inches
5cm	2 inches
8cm	3¼ inches
10cm	4 inches
20cm	8 inches
25cm	10 inches
30cm	12 inches

ACKNOWLEDGEMENTS

To my mum, Sandra, and sister, Nina: thank you for showing me, by example, what a great mother is. Your loving, firm but fair – and extremely funny – ways throughout my life have moulded me into the woman and mother I am today. If I can be even half the mum to Mia that you've been to me, I know I'm doing it right. I love you both.

To Gorka, for giving me the most precious gift I never knew I needed. Mia has your stubbornness, which makes me laugh daily. I love watching the bond you two share. She's incredibly lucky to have such a wonderful Papa.

To my agent Becca and all the team at BBM, for believing in me with every opportunity that's handed to me – including this second book! You really are the Dream Team!

To Olly Foster for once again helping me create a challenging yet achievable plan, and for always prioritising my health above everything else. Your knowledge of all things health and fitness is invaluable. And to Nick Mitchell, Evil Steve (who isn't evil at all) and all the team at UP Fitness Manchester for providing my shoot location. If Carlsberg did gyms... Ultimate Performance would be it! You guys are incredible, and I always feel welcome in your gyms.

To Jo Usmar, for once more understanding from the off how I wanted this book to be. Your passion and enthusiasm for wanting to help women feel their best and keep it real is infectious. I'll miss our long chats about literally everything!

Headline Books – I cannot thank you enough! It's because of Lindsey and the team that this book is here. From that first email to a group Zoom, to ideas and shared stories,and from shoot locations and food pictures – to this! I'm so thankful to you all, and I'm so proud to have my second book in your safe hands. You are all remarkable.

To David Cummings and the photography team. They say to never work with dogs or children, and on the shoot days, we had both! Thank you for capturing such lovely memories and moments.

To my wonderful family and friends, for always filling my life with such fun, laughter and adventures – and for loving Mia so much. 'GanGan Peter', you are Mia's favourite (sorry Mum! LOL!)

To my dogs, Norman and Ollie: you taught me how to be a dog mum for eight years before I had Mia, and you're both the best 'big brothers'. I'll never forget the day we brought Mia home to meet you both.

And last but by no means least, to Mia Louise Marquez. Beautiful Mia. My reason for everything. You've changed my life in ways I never knew possible, and because of you, I now know what unconditional love is. If you ever need anything in life – a chat, a cuddle, an ex's car scratched (kidding!! LOL!) – Mum's got you covered.

I love you xx

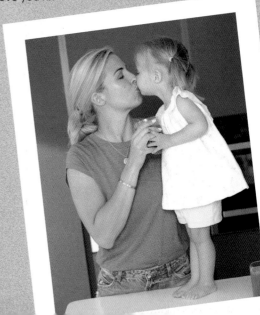

First published in 2022
by Headline Home
An imprint of Headline Publishing Group

1

Cataloguing in Publication Data is available from the
British Library

Trade paperback ISBN 9781472283801

eISBN 9781472283825

Headline's policy is to use papers that are natural,
renewable and recyclable products and
made from wood grown in sustainable forests. The
logging and manufacturing processes are
expected to conform to the environmental
regulations of the country of origin.

Printed and bound in Italy by LEGO S.p.A
Colour reproduction by ALTA London

HEADLINE PUBLISHING GROUP
An Hachette UK Company
Carmelite House
50 Victoria Embankment
London EC4Y 0DZ

www.headline.co.uk
www.hachette.co.uk

Commissioning Editor: Lindsey Evans
Designed by Nikki Dupin, Studio Nic & Lou
Food photography: Dan Jones
Fitness and lifestyle photography: David Cummings*
Fitness advisor: Olly Foster
Nutritionist: Laura Matthews
Food styling: Christina Mackenzie
Food styling assistants: Bee Berrie, Axel McHugh
and Lizzie Evans
Prop styling (food): Charlie Phillips
Prop styling (fitness and lifestyle): Andie Redman
Hair and make-up: Heather Marnie
Project editors: Kate Miles and Tara O'Sullivan
Proofreader: Claire Rogers
Indexer: Caroline Wilding

* images on pages 13, 18, 30, 35 and 39 provided by
the author.

Gym workouts shot at Ultimate Performance
Personal Training
(www.ultimateperformance.com)